NATURAL CURES AND GENTLE MEDICINES

That Unleash Your Body's Healing Power

Publisher's Note

This book is for information only. It does not constitute medical advice and should not be construed as such. We cannot guarantee the safety or effectiveness of any drug, treatment, or advice mentioned. Some of these tips may not be effective for everyone.

A good doctor is the best judge of what medical treatment may be needed for certain conditions and diseases. We recommend in all cases that you contact your personal doctor or health care provider before taking or discontinuing any medications, or before treating yourself in any way.

FC&A
103 Clover Green
Peachtree City, GA 30269

Produced by the staff of FC&A

Distributed to the trade by National Book Network

Cover Images: © 1992, 1994, 1995, 1996
PhotoDisc, Inc.

Do not be anxious about anything, but in everything, by prayer and petition, with thanksgiving, present your requests to God. And the peace of God, which transcends all understanding, will guard your hearts and your minds in Christ Jesus.

Philippians 4:6-7 (NIV)

The fear of the Lord is the beginning of wisdom; A good understanding have all those who do His commandments; His praise endures forever.

Psalm 111:10

Table of Contents

Cholesterol

Chronic Pain

Colds and Flu

Colon Cancer

Constipation

Depression

Diabetes

Introduction

Modern medicine is truly miraculous. In this century, particularly in the last few decades, doctors and scientists have discovered medicines and procedures that have cured many diseases and enabled people to live longer.

However, these advances don't come without a price, and the cost is more than just monetary. Modern drugs have saved many lives, but they have also taken lives as well. According to a study published in the *Journal of the American Medical Association,* more than 100,000 people every year die from adverse drug reactions. That makes it between the fourth and sixth leading cause of death in the United States.

Surgery also may save your life, but many needless surgeries are performed every year. One study found that heart patients who underwent bypass surgery were significantly more likely to die or have another heart attack as those who were treated without surgery.

So how do you know when you should take advantage of modern medical technology and when you should choose an alternative? Your doctor is a great source of guidance, of course, but he needs your help to understand your specific health problems. No one knows your body better than you do, and the more you learn how to take care of it, the better you can control your own health.

Buying this book is an important first step in learning to deal with the most common health problems today. *Natural Cures and Gentle Medicines That Work Better Than Dangerous Drugs or Risky Surgery* provides you with the knowledge you need to make decisions about your own health.

We gathered information from reputable medical journals all over the world and interviewed dozens of experts to compile an encyclopedia of the latest health news and knowledge just for you. You'll find practical tips for easy things you can do at home to keep every part of your body strong and vital, from your bones to your brain.

The book is organized alphabetically by condition to make it easy for you to locate your area of concern or interest. If you have a health problem — from acne to heart disease to warts — you'll find information to help you deal with it in *Natural Cures and Gentle Medicines.* If you're healthy as a horse, and would like to stay that way, you can also find the latest preventive knowledge within these pages. Either way, you're sure to discover something useful for yourself or a loved one.

We're glad you've trusted us to provide you with reliable medical information that can help you enjoy a longer and more fulfilling life. Use it in good health!

The Editors of FC&A

Acne

Clearing up acne myths

Slumber parties, geometry, prom, summer camp — and acne. Manager meetings, car payments, PTA — and acne. You don't have to be a teenager to get hit with pimples and blackheads. A recent survey found that 81 percent of people with acne were 15 to 44 years old. If you find yourself over 30 and battling breakouts, don't despair. First, learn the truth behind acne myths — then form a plan of attack.

Myth #1: Acne will go away on its own. Some people think if you leave pimples alone, they'll eventually go away. While it's true many breakouts will heal, if you treat acne right away, you're less likely to suffer from both emotional and physical scarring.

If you're looking for a treatment without chemicals, try a natural antibacterial from Australia called tea tree oil. A 5 percent tea tree oil gel was tested against the popular acne treatment benzoyl peroxide lotion, and it came out a winner. The tea tree oil reduced breakouts just as effectively as the benzoyl peroxide but with fewer side effects. Look for tea tree oil lotion and soap at your local bath and body shop.

Myth #2: Acne is caused by dirt. Pimples form when oil from overactive oil glands mixes with dead skin cells and plugs up your pores. To keep your face clean, wash it twice a day with mild, unscented soap and warm water. Scrubbing your face constantly and using harsh soaps will not wash away your acne. In fact, it can make the condition worse.

Here's a natural cleanser you can make at home. Heat some lemon juice until barely warm and add two egg whites. Whip this mixture until it forms a thick paste. Store any unused cleanser in the refrigerator.

Myth #3: Acne is caused by the foods you eat. Although lots of healthy foods, like fresh fruits and vegetables, are important to healthy skin, eating chocolate and pizza will not cause acne. Just eat a balanced diet and drink lots of water.

Myth #4: Sunlight helps acne. Tanning or using a sunlamp on your face may hide your acne, but only temporarily. The long-term effects of sun exposure, aging and skin cancer, far outweigh any immediate benefits. Use a sunscreen, but choose one that's oil-free.

Myth #5: Squeezing pimples helps them heal faster. The exact opposite is true. You are much more likely to cause redness and swelling, even scarring, by picking. If you must do something, try one of these natural treatments for breakouts:

- ▶ wrap an ice cube in a soft cloth and hold it to the blemish for a few minutes every hour

- ▶ rub a peeled slice of potato gently over freshly washed skin

- ▶ dab a small amount of toothpaste on the blemish at night just before bed

- ▶ lay a lemon slice over your breakouts for a few minutes

Here's how the experts treat acne

Most acne is caused by overactive oil glands in your face, upper back, and chest. If you decide to seek help from a dermatologist, he may prescribe one or more of these products, depending on the severity of your acne.

Peeling agents. These include lotions or ointments you apply in a thin film. They will dry your skin and often cause redness. If you suffer from mild acne, your dermatologist will most likely recommend starting with one of these products.

- ▶ Benzoyl peroxide (Benoxyl, Oxy 10) is available over-the-counter or in stronger doses through a prescription. It helps reduce acne-causing bacteria and unblocks clogged pores.

- ▶ Tretinoin, retinoic acid, or vitamin A acid (Renova, Retin-A) prevent pimples and blackheads from forming. They will make your skin very sensitive to sunlight. To reduce skin irritation, avoid using other drying lotions, medicated cleansers and make-up, or skin products containing alcohol.

▶ Salicylic acid, sulfur, or resorcinol help remove dead skin cells. You'll find these ingredients in many over-the-counter acne products.

Topical antibiotics. These creams or ointments reduce the amount of bacteria on your skin or suppress the bacteria in your oil glands. You may use these alone or with other products, such as oral antibiotics.

They can cause redness, tingling, or stinging and often dry out your skin. Some topical antibiotics may seem to make your skin oilier. If you use them with other acne treatments or with soaps, cosmetics, or shaving products containing alcohol, your skin may become irritated. Topical antibiotics will make your skin more sensitive to the sun.

Some examples are azelaic acid cream, clindamycin phosphate, erythromycin, metronidazole, and tetracycline hydrochloride.

Oral medications. These drugs are prescribed for cases of acne that don't clear up with milder treatments. You can use these alone or along with topical products.

▶ Tetracycline hydrochloride (Achromycin) is an antibiotic for moderate acne. This drug can make your skin very sensitive to the sun. Other antibiotics in the tetracycline family are doxycycline hydrochloride and minocycline hydrochloride.

▶ Birth control pills are often prescribed for women with acne. They decrease the effects of male hormones, which stimulate oil glands.

▶ Isotretinoin (Accutane) is prescribed for severe acne. It shrinks oil glands and changes the consistency of the oil produced, making it less likely to block your pores. Talk with your doctor about the possible side effects of isotretinoin. They include depression, headaches, fatigue, dry eyes and lips, extreme dry skin, and high cholesterol and triglyceride levels. This drug can also cause severe birth defects if taken during pregnancy.

Allergies

A-plus ways to avoid air-borne irritants

If the very air around you seems to be your enemy, you probably suffer from allergies, but you can take comfort in knowing that you are not alone. It is the most common chronic disease, accounting for one out of every 40 doctor visits.

Hay fever, or allergic rhinitis, is a seasonal condition if you're allergic to pollen, but it is a year-round problem if you're allergic to dust, mold, or animal dander.

Whenever these tiny air-borne allergens get into your system, they cause the lining of your nose and sinuses to swell. This can result in sneezing, stuffy or runny nose, itching, coughing, and sore throat.

It may be hard to fight something so small you can't even see it, but it's not impossible. Here are some tips for keeping your allergies under control.

Use the sun to battle dust mites. Dust mites are tiny insects that live in bedding, carpets, and mattresses. They eat dead, sloughed-off human skin cells and give off waste material that can trigger allergic reactions. Whenever you change your sheets or vacuum, this waste material blows around in the air for about 30 minutes, and inhaling it can set off an episode of sniffling, sneezing, and coughing.

Sunlight may help you combat those pesky bugs. A study in Australia found that leaving mite-infested rugs outside for four hours on a hot, sunny day killed 100 percent of mites and their eggs. This would probably work for bedding, curtains, and pillows as well.

Try tannic acid. For carpets and rugs you can't take outside, a tannic acid solution may be just what you need. Researchers found that one type of this solution, Allersearch ADS, reduced dust mites in carpet by up to 92 percent.

6

Control the mold. Try to keep your house as dry as possible to limit the growth of mold. Check areas that tend to be damp, like under sinks, and around toilets, tubs, and washing machines, and wipe these places down with bleach and water. Houseplants and aquariums can also harbor mold. If you must have houseplants, you can buy mold retardants from your local nursery.

Stay inside. If you're allergic to pollen, staying inside whenever pollen levels are high may help. Spring and fall are the seasons most likely to cause problems. Grass and tree pollen make spring a season of sniffling, and in the fall, ragweed starts the sneezing anew. Pollen levels also tend to be highest in the morning hours, so staying inside until afternoon may help.

Wear a mask. If you have to work in your yard, wear a mask that covers your nose and mouth, especially while cutting grass. It will block out at least some of the allergens. If you're allergic to dust, wear a mask whenever you have to dust or vacuum your house.

Shower up. After outdoor activities, take a quick shower to remove any pollen residue from your skin and hair. Your hair can harbor a lot of pollen, especially if it's long, so it's particularly important to shampoo before going to bed.

Close your windows. Make sure your bedroom windows are closed at night to keep allergens out and help you rest easier.

Use air-conditioning. Air-conditioners reduce the humidity and pollen levels in your house and allow you to keep your windows closed and still remain comfortable in hot weather.

Keep pets outside. Pet dander (dead skin cells) is a major cause of allergies. The fleas on your pet may also aggravate your hay fever. If you have furry or feathered pets that you can't bear to part with, try to keep them outside. If that's not possible, make sure they are bathed often, and use something to control the fleas.

Ditch the aerosols. Use pump-spray products whenever possible because aerosol sprays may irritate your airways.

Cover bedding. Enclosing pillows and mattresses in zippered vinyl coverings can help keep dust mites from collecting.

Unclutter your life. You may be emotionally attached to all those knickknacks, but the more items in your house that can collect dust, the worse your allergies may get. Venetian blinds and chandeliers are other household dust-collectors that you should eliminate from your home.

Shoot down allergens with allergy shots

If you have allergies, keeping your "triggers" at bay can be quite a job. You may not want to take medications because of their undesirable side effects, such as drowsiness.

But if you're like thousands of other Americans, you may not even know about an effective alternative — allergy shots.

One reason many people don't take advantage of this treatment may be its name — immunotherapy. The American Academy of Allergy, Asthma, and Immunology (ACAAI) believes people are confused and perhaps even frightened by the term. The group recommends that doctors start calling the allergy shots "vaccinations" instead of "immunotherapy" to make people feel more comfortable.

Allergy vaccines require that you first be tested for specific allergens. Then your doctor injects you with small amounts of the purified allergen, gradually increasing the dosage over time until your immunity is built up. The process usually continues for several years, but if you suffer from severe allergies, you'll see a dramatic improvement in your life.

Lift your glass to allergy relief

The birds are singing and flowers are in bloom. But the minute you step outside to enjoy the beauty of spring, the sniffling and sneezing start. Once again, pollen forces you inside to watch the world through your windows.

Relief for your distress could be nearer than you think — as close, in fact, as your kitchen sink. Your allergy symptoms may really be a sign of thirst.

That's the opinion of Fereydoon Batmanghelidj, M.D., author of the book *Your Body's Many Cries for Water*. He suggests you prevent the discomforts of allergies by drinking more water.

The substance that regulates the way your body uses water is called histamine. If you don't drink enough water and become dehydrated, your body wants to correct the problem. It does this by releasing an extra dose of histamine that has been stored for other uses.

This causes watery eyes and a runny nose. You may be tempted to take an antihistamine to dry them up, but this medication can produce some unpleasant side effects — like dry mouth, drowsiness, headache, and nausea.

In fact, Batmanghelidj believes antihistamines may be dangerous because they interfere with the body's natural attempts to correct the underlying problem. Instead of popping a pill, try these tips from Dr. B. (as he calls himself on his web site at www.watercure.com).

Drink six to eight 8-ounce glasses of water a day. That's pure water — not alcohol, tea, coffee, or cola. Limit orange juice to one or two glasses a day, and don't include it in your water count. "The potassium content of orange juice is high," says Dr. B. "High loads of potassium in the body can promote more than the usual histamine production."

Open your kitchen cabinet, not your medicine cabinet. Reach for something less expensive than the antihistamine you buy at the drugstore. "Salt," says Batmanghelidj, "is a natural antihistamine. People with allergies should begin to increase their salt intake to prevent excess histamine production."

Be patient. You'll probably find it takes one to four weeks before you start noticing a change. Don't try to speed up the process by drinking more than the recommended six to eight glasses of water.

"First and foremost," says Dr. B., "do not imagine you could reverse the situation if you now drown yourself in water. Not so!" It takes a while for your cells to soak up the water and rehydrate your body.

Most people, according to Dr. B., have lost the ability to tell when they are thirsty. Once your body adjusts to having plenty of water, you should notice your natural thirst returning. You may then find you want more than eight glasses a day. That's okay — but let it happen naturally.

Drink the most around meal times. While you should drink water any time you're thirsty, Dr. B. suggests you drink one glass one-half hour before meals. Have another glass two and a half hours after each meal. Add two more glasses around your heaviest meal or before you go to bed.

All this water keeps your blood from becoming too concentrated after you've digested a lot of food. Without enough water flowing through your system, the thicker blood pulls water from the cells around it, and you can become dehydrated. And, as Dr. B. points out, allergies are just one of several conditions caused or aggravated by dehydration.

Tap a handy water supply. Water from your kitchen sink may be your best source of drinking water. If you depend on bottled water, you may run out. You are then likely to wait longer and not drink enough.

If there's a chance your water is contaminated, have it tested. You may need to install a water filter. If a chlorine taste puts you off, let some water sit in an open pitcher until the chlorine evaporates.

Don't let pollen or other allergens spoil your fun. Just sit back and sip those extra glasses of water. Before long, you'll be able to breathe easy when you go outside.

Are you allergic to sex?

It's true — some women actually have such an unusual allergy. These cases typically are not allergies to the act of sex itself, but to some element of sex — most frequently, semen. A relatively small percentage of women are allergic to the proteins found in semen, and this sensitivity can cause a wide range of symptoms.

Although not very common, sexual allergies can be quite severe. "It's rare," says Dr. Jonathan Bernstein of the University of Cincinnati College of Medicine, who has researched sexual allergies for more than 10 years. "But it's also hard to get reliable figures on something this personal. My best guess is that one women in a thousand is affected by this problem."

Reactions to semen might be as simple as mild vaginal pain, swelling and itching, or as dramatic as outbreaks of hives and difficulty breathing. But if you are the unfortunate victim of this type of allergy, it doesn't mean the end of your sex life.

Bernstein and his colleagues at the University of Cincinnati have developed methods for the successful treatment of such allergies using vaccines, allowing affected people to return to their normal sex lives. Doctors working on the same problem in California have devised a cream that, when used before sex, has been shown to completely prevent reactions even in highly allergic women.

The problem with the vaccinations is that they are not cheap. "It's getting better," says Bernstein. "We've been able to shrink the cost of treatment from $5,000 to about $2,000. But for most people, that's still not practical." What is practical, though — and cheap — is a seemingly obvious choice that most people apparently don't think about.

"You'd be surprised," says Bernstein, "at how many people don't even think to use a condom. Or use it wrong. It's cheap, it's safe, it's practical, and as long as you use it properly, it works." If you know you're allergic to semen, simply using a condom during sex can prevent contact and reactions. "From a practical standpoint, it's still probably your best bet," he says.

There are also drug treatments available for dealing with this problem, and your doctor can help you decide which of these options is right for you. So if you are having difficulty or experiencing pain before, during, or after sex, don't put it off — see your doctor right away.

Alzheimer's Disease

10 ways to spot Alzheimer's early

Every time you forget where you left your car keys, do you think you're getting Alzheimer's? You're probably overly concerned, but you should be aware of the risk factors of the disease. You are more likely to get Alzheimer's if you're female, over 65, have a family history of the disease, have Down's syndrome, or have had a serious head injury in the past.

Detecting Alzheimer's early may help slow its progress, so you should be aware of these early warning signs that you or a loved one may have the disease.

Forgetfulness. The most well-known signal that you might have Alzheimer's is simply forgetfulness. While it's normal to forget names or lose your keys once in a while, frequent forgetfulness may be a red flag. The classic example is that it is normal to forget your keys, but if you can't remember what the keys are for, it's time to worry.

Speech problems. Sometimes a word is on the tip of your tongue, but you just can't get it out. Everyone has that experience occasionally, but if you often have trouble with simple words, or your speech isn't understandable, you may have a problem.

Misplacing things. Some people lose track of their keys or the TV remote almost every day. But finding lost items in a strange place, like the microwave or the refrigerator, should be cause for concern.

Personality changes. Everyone goes through changes in their lives. Some people become more laid-back and relaxed as they age, while others seem to turn into grumpy old men and women. However, Alzheimer's can cause profound personality changes, turning a calm, sweet person into someone who's frightened, paranoid, or confused.

Loss of judgment. You may think young people show poor judgment in their choice of clothes, but if you can't judge what clothing is appropriate for you to wear, you may be the one with a problem. For example, if you put your socks on your hands, or wear shorts when it's snowing, you have lost your ability to judge.

Loss of interest. Everyone can lose interest in a slow-paced movie, but when you aren't interested in all the things that used to bring you pleasure, like hobbies, that's a little more serious.

Problems with familiar tasks. Busy people often are distracted and may forget to finish something they started. Someone with Alzheimer's might prepare a meal and not only forget to serve it, but not remember she even made it in the first place. Or she may have problems remembering how to prepare the meal at all.

Mood swings. Although most people are moody sometimes, going from one extreme to the other rapidly for no apparent reason is cause for concern.

Disorientation. If you get lost in a strange city, no one would accuse you of having Alzheimer's. If you get lost in your own neighborhood, that's another story. Place or time disorientation is an early symptom of Alzheimer's. If you easily forget what day it is or how to get to a familiar place, you should see a doctor.

Trouble "adding it up." Maybe math was your worst subject in school. Still, if doing simple math problems suddenly becomes more difficult, you may have a problem yourself. Math requires abstract thinking, connecting symbols (numbers) with a meaning. Abstract thinking is one of the first skills you lose with Alzheimer's.

Getting to the root of Alzheimer's

It seems as if every day someone comes up with a new theory about what causes Alzheimer's disease (AD). Although no one has yet pinpointed a specific cause, researchers continue their efforts to understand the roots of the problem. And they have come up with several promising possibilities that may help you avoid this memory-robbing disease.

Small strokes may be harmful. Strokes can kill or paralyze you, but new research finds that even minor strokes that don't cause such obvious damage can contribute to Alzheimer's.

Researchers found that if you have even one or two small strokes in certain regions of your brain, you may dramatically increase your risk of AD. They studied more than 100 women for the tell-tale lesions of Alzheimer's disease. Among women who had many lesions, those who had the small strokes were more than 20 times as likely to have dementia as women who had never had a stroke.

Certain jobs can be risky. People who have jobs that require tools with electric motors may be more likely to develop AD. These tools can give off electro-magnetic fields (EMFs) that may contribute to the development of the disease.

Seamstresses, dressmakers, and tailors, who work huddled over electric sewing machines, are three times more likely to get Alzheimer's than most people. The only occupations with a greater risk of AD are electric power line workers and welders.

Environmental hazards are a gamble. People who are exposed to solvent solutions in their jobs, like painters, are more likely to get Alzheimer's. And some research indicates that pesticides, like DDT, may also contribute to the disease. If you have to deal with chemical solvents or pesticides on the job or at home, handle them carefully.

Viral/bacterial link is possible. Some scientists think an infection of the brain may lead to Alzheimer's. This infection could be caused by a virus or by bacteria. When scientists examined the brains of people who had died of Alzheimer's, they found a bacterium called *Chlamydia pneumoniae* in areas damaged by Alzheimer's. However, they still don't know whether the bacteria might have led to Alzheimer's or entered the brain after it was damaged.

Common minerals may be toxic. Small amounts of certain trace elements, such as zinc and aluminum, have shown up in the brain tissue of people with Alzheimer's disease. Researchers aren't sure whether these substances caused the disease or resulted from it.

► **Zinc.** If you have risk factors for Alzheimer's, you might want to check the label on any supplements you're taking. Research finds that large amounts of the mineral zinc can cause plaques similar to the ones found in the brains of people with Alzheimer's. It is unknown whether excess zinc can actually cause Alzheimer's, but it might be wise to limit your intake to no more than the recommended dietary allowance of 8 to 11 mg a day.

► **Aluminum.** This mineral is one of the most controversial risk factors for Alzheimer's. You can get it from many sources, including aluminum cookware and anti-perspirant, but it is also commonly found in your water supply. Experts still disagree about whether it contributes to AD, but most don't think that aluminum in your drinking water poses a serious threat to your memories. If you want to be cautious, however, you can have your water tested, or just buy bottled water.

Amino acid may increase risk. The amino acid homocysteine has been associated with an increased risk of heart disease and stroke and now has also been linked to Alzheimer's. Researchers have found that people with Alzheimer's are more likely to have elevated levels of homocysteine in their blood.

More research is needed to determine whether the excess homocysteine may be a cause or a result of the disease. But if it does turn out to be a factor, that could actually be good news. Researchers have found that B vitamins, particularly folic acid, effectively reduce homocysteine levels.

7 simple steps to prevent Alzheimer's

One out of every 10 people over the age of 65 has Alzheimer's disease (AD). And an estimated 14 million Americans will develop it by the middle of the next century unless a cure is found. If you want to avoid becoming an Alzheimer's statistic, you need to start on the road to prevention now.

Take an aspirin and hang onto your memories. Some doctors think inflamed brain tissue might contribute to Alzheimer's. That would mean NSAIDs (non-steroidal anti-inflammatories) like aspirin or ibuprofen might help prevent or treat the condition by reducing swelling.

Research indicates this could be true. One study of 50 elderly twins found that the twin who used NSAIDs was less likely to get Alzheimer's, or developed it later in life, than the twin who didn't use NSAIDs.

These promising and inexpensive remedies may be just what you need to stem the tide of Alzheimer's disease. However, taking too many anti-inflammatory drugs may cause side effects, mainly stomach irritation or bleeding, so talk to your doctor before starting any treatment.

Slow down AD the "E-Z" way. A simple vitamin may help you buy some time before Alzheimer's steals your health. This miracle vitamin, which a recent study found can slow the progression of AD, is the highly touted antioxidant, vitamin E.

Researchers divided people with Alzheimer's into four groups. They gave one group 2,000 IU of vitamin E daily. Another group took selegiline, a drug used to treat Parkinson's disease. The other groups got either a combination of vitamin E and selegiline or a placebo.

The people who took either the vitamin E or the selegiline were able to care for themselves longer, and delayed entering a nursing home by about seven months, compared to the people who got the placebo.

A 2,000-IU dose is much larger than that found in supplements and could cause bleeding problems, so talk to your doctor before taking vitamin E. A simple multivitamin that includes this powerful antioxidant may be all you need to help you maintain your independence longer.

Discover a natural way to "leaf" AD behind. An herb that supposedly improves your memory should surely help combat a disease that slowly drains your memories out of you, shouldn't it?

According to new research, it does. A study found that an extract made from the nuts, leaves, and branches of the ginkgo biloba plant may slow down the course of Alzheimer's disease for some people. In the study, a substantial number of people with AD who took the extract delayed the progression of the disease by six months to one year.

This effect is about the same as two prescription drugs approved by the FDA for treating Alzheimer's (Aricept and Cognex) and produced no significant side effects.

Stop smoking and snuff out Alzheimer's. You know smoking is bad for your lungs, but what does it do to your brain? Earlier studies came to the surprising conclusion that smoking may protect you against Alzheimer's. These reports were based on the fact that more Alzheimer's victims are non-smokers.

But a recent study found that smoking actually increases your chances of Alzheimer's and other forms of dementia. More than 6,000 people ages 55 and over were followed for two years. Almost 150 people developed Alzheimer's or other dementia during that period. According to researchers, smoking doubled the risk of the disease.

Why the difference in results? It may be that non-smokers live longer and, therefore, have more time to develop the disease. Smoking is the number one cause of premature death in developed countries like the United States. Since Alzheimer's strikes mostly older people, smokers may not be affected simply because they die from lung cancer or other causes before Alzheimer's can develop.

Look to hormones for help. Women are twice as likely to get Alzheimer's disease as men. However, a large study conducted by the National Institute on Aging found that postmenopausal women who used estrogen were 54 percent less likely to get Alzheimer's than women who had never taken estrogen.

Another study found that estrogen may also help ease the symptoms of AD. Women who already had the disease were treated with estrogen. Within a week, these women showed signs of improvement, while women who didn't get estrogen did not.

Learn something new every day. Education may be the key to success, but it also may be the key to sidestepping Alzheimer's. Recent studies have found that the more education you have, the lower your risk of AD.

Education may protect your brain indirectly by making you more likely to eat better, exercise, and obtain good medical care. However, the most important thing it does is to increase connections between your brain cells. Alzheimer's disease destroys the lines of communication, called synapses, between your brain cells. Every time you learn something new, you build new connections, thus strengthening your memory and fighting off AD.

To keep Alzheimer's at bay, try to learn something new every day. A crossword puzzle, word game, picture puzzle, or interesting new book will help keep those synapses snapping.

Angina

Easing the ache of angina

It's finally spring, and you're working in your yard for the first time in months. You actually enjoy the hard work until your chest begins to feel a little tight and then becomes downright painful. Whether it's the first time you've felt angina pain, or it's an old familiar feeling, it helps to know how best to deal with the problem.

Angina occurs when part of your heart muscle isn't getting enough blood and, therefore, not enough oxygen. This usually happens when your heart's need for oxygen increases suddenly, like during exercise. Stress, eating a heavy meal, extreme heat or cold, and smoking cigarettes can also trigger this heart problem.

Exercise in moderation. It may not seem logical to recommend exercise to someone with angina when exercise is the main trigger. But regular, moderate exercise will keep your heart strong and build healthier blood vessels to carry oxygen. Work with your doctor to develop an exercise program that's right for you. Walking is usually the recommended exercise, beginning with short, five-minute walks and gradually increasing until you're walking for 30 minutes, at least two or three days a week.

Kick the habit. If you smoke and you have angina, you have another excellent reason to kick the habit. Next time you start to light up, think about how much your chest hurts during an angina attack, and instead, get some help in quitting. Your doctor can recommend strategies to help you stop smoking.

Lessen stress. Everyone has some stress in their lives, but if you can learn to handle it better, you may improve your angina. Think about what types of situations cause you tension, and try to avoid them. Of course, it's impossible to avoid all stressful situations, so try to learn techniques for dealing with stress. (See the *Stress* chapter for more information.)

Limit fat and lose weight. Too much fat in your diet and on your body contributes to clogged arteries, which can lead to angina. Many people find that when they shed those extra pounds, their angina disappears.

Take an aspirin. You may know that daily aspirin can help prevent heart attacks and strokes, but guess what — it may also help lessen angina. The recommended dosage for angina is 75-325 mg daily, but ask your doctor before beginning aspirin therapy.

Keep your nitro handy. If you've been diagnosed with angina, your doctor may have prescribed nitroglycerine. However, it won't do you any good if it's sitting in your medicine cabinet when you have an angina attack on the golf course. Keep it with you at all times.

Control blood pressure. The lower your blood pressure, the lighter your heart's workload, and the less oxygen it needs. Watch your fat and salt intake, and avoid over-the-counter medications that may raise your blood pressure. If your doctor has prescribed medicine for lowering your blood pressure, be sure you take it as directed. (See the *High Blood Pressure* chapter for more information.)

Eat small meals. Eating a heavy meal can bring on an angina attack because too much of your blood flow is directed to digesting your food. Eating smaller, more frequent meals can help you avoid that.

Learning more about angina will help you understand and control it better. For more information, contact:

▶ American Heart Association, 7272 Greenville Ave., Dallas, TX, 75231, phone: (800) AHA-USA1

▶ National Heart, Lung, and Blood Institute Information Center, P.O. Box 30105, Bethesda, MD, 20824-0105, phone: (301) 592-8573

▶ The Mended Hearts, Inc., 7272 Greenville Ave., Dallas, TX, 75231-4596, phone: (214) 706-1442

Amazing new angina treatments

Lifestyle changes can sometimes ease angina symptoms, but when just walking up a hill becomes an ordeal requiring several stops and nitroglycerine tablets, you may need serious medical treatment. If that happens, you should know that new options are now available.

Although many factors can trigger an attack of angina, the real culprit behind the pain is usually fatty deposits clogging your arteries. This blockage in your arteries makes it harder for blood to get to your heart. The conventional treatments doctors usually recommend to clear those blocked arteries are balloon angioplasty or bypass surgery.

Angioplasty involves inserting a balloon-tipped tube into the artery with blockage and then expanding it, pushing the walls of the artery outward. However, about 30 percent of angioplasties fail because the artery closes back up. Bypass surgery can also fail, and it is a highly traumatic surgery to endure.

Luckily, researchers are constantly discovering more options in angina treatment. Some exciting new techniques can even help your body perform a kind of natural bypass — growing new blood vessels to replace the clogged ones.

Bypass old arteries with new genes. In a technique called gene therapy, doctors inject the gene coding for a protein called vascular endothelial growth factor, or VEGF, into your heart. Amazingly, this protein encourages new blood vessels to grow from existing ones. These new vessels bypass the clogged ones and carry more oxygen-rich blood to your heart muscle. And the really good news is that they are less likely to clog up in the future than your original arteries.

One potential side effect is the growth of hemangiomas, which are masses of abnormal blood vessel tissue. One study on rats found that some did develop hemangiomas, but so far that hasn't been seen in humans. The main problem is that sometimes the treatment just doesn't work, although the success rate has been fairly high. Out of the first 82 patients to receive gene therapy, 60 of them showed signs of new vessel growth.

The treatment is still considered experimental, but these results are promising. It is far less traumatic to the patient than bypass surgery and will probably cost much less, which is good news for angina sufferers.

Stimulate new vessels with inflatable cuffs. A new treatment called external counterpulsation (EECP) may stimulate new blood vessel growth much like gene therapy but without the injections.

In EECP, inflatable cuffs are placed on your calves, thighs, and buttocks. These then inflate and deflate, driving the blood flow up toward your heart. This causes small vessels around your heart to expand and carry more blood. After several treatments, the small vessels become permanent suppliers to your heart.

Your doctor may not be familiar with EECP, but it is available at these major medical centers: Mayo Clinic, Rochester, N.Y.; Ochsner Foundation Hospital, New Orleans, La.; University of California's San Diego and San Francisco medical centers; and medical centers at the University of Florida, University of Pittsburgh, and University of Virginia.

Drill your heart for immediate relief. In this technique, called transmyocardial revascularization or TMR, doctors use lasers to drill tiny holes in the muscle of your heart. It sounds scary, but there's no need to worry. The holes close up on the outside of your heart almost immediately, while the channels created by the laser remain open on the inside of the muscle.

These channels fill with blood that bring much-needed oxygen to your heart. That's probably why people often experience immediate relief from angina with this method. It definitely provides short-term relief, but it may work long term as well. One study found that after almost three years, people who had been treated with TMR were maintaining their improvement.

These unusual treatments may make open-heart surgery unnecessary for many heart patients. If your doctor recommends angioplasty or bypass surgery for your angina, ask him about these new options before making a decision.

Boost your medicine's healing power

In comedy, timing is everything. When it comes to taking your medication, timing may also be important, and the results of poor timing could be no laughing matter, especially when it comes to your heart.

Your body has certain rhythms, which means your medication can affect you differently at different times of the day. If you take your medicine at the right time, you may actually boost its effectiveness and increase your chances of feeling better. On the other hand, if you take it at the wrong time, you may prevent the medication from working at full strength and miss getting its full benefits.

The first hour or two after arising is the most likely time for you to have a heart attack or stroke. If you suffer from angina, it is also the time most likely to have an attack of chest pain. Most angina patients tend to feel worse in the morning and gradually get better as the day progresses.

There are several possible reasons for this. Blood volume to your heart tends to decrease in the morning, blood tends to clot more, and your arteries are narrower. Your blood pressure also naturally falls at night as your body prepares for sleep, and it rises about 20 percent right after you wake up.

Because of this, some angina medication is designed to be extended release, so that if you take it at night, it is working at its best in the morning, when you need it most.

Blood pressure medication, however, may work better if you take it as soon as you wake up, instead of after you shower, shave, dress, and cook breakfast.

Heart conditions aren't the only ones that may benefit from timing medication. In one study, children with leukemia who took their maintenance medication in the evening were three times less likely to experience a relapse than children who took their medication in the morning.

Other conditions that may benefit from timing your medication include:

▶ **Asthma.** Some drugs used to treat asthma work better when taken in the late afternoon instead of in the morning.

▶ **Arthritis.** If your arthritis bothers you most in the morning, nonsteroidal anti-inflammatory drugs (NSAIDs) work better if taken in the evening. If you have more pain in the evening, your NSAID will work better if you take it around noon.

▶ **Ulcers.** Ulcer medications like cimetidine (Tagamet) and famotidine (Pepcid) work best if taken once a day with your evening meal.

Whenever your doctor writes you a prescription, be sure to ask him if there is a particular time of day that is best to take your medication. You may even want to set a daily alarm so you can take advantage of the extra "healing power" good timing will provide.

Cracking the prescription code

When your doctor writes you a prescription, does it look like Greek to you? Actually, it's Latin. Most directions on your prescription are based on a Latin word or phrase. If you'd like to make sense of it all, here are a few common abbreviations you might see.

Abbreviation	*Meaning*
a.c.	before meals
ad lib	as much as wanted
b.i.d.	twice a day
h.	hour
h.s.	at bedtime
p.	after
p.c.	after meals
p.o.	by mouth
p.r.n.	as necessary
q.	every
q.4 h.	every four hours
q.d.	every day
q.i.d.	four times a day
q.o.d.	every other day
Rx	prescription
stat.	immediately
t.i.d.	three times a day

Arthritis

Tame arthritis pain by changing what you eat

If you have an ache in your stomach, your first thought is likely to be, "It must be something I ate." You probably wouldn't associate an ache in your joints with your diet, but research indicates that what you eat may indeed make your arthritis better or worse. To find relief from the pain, try changing your diet.

Dish up some fish. If joint pain makes it difficult for you to climb out of bed in the morning, maybe you should eat more fish. Several studies have found that omega-3 fatty acids, which are found in fatty fish, can help relieve some of the joint pain and stiffness caused by arthritis.

Eating fish may even help protect you from developing arthritis. One large study found that women who ate at least one to two servings of fish each week were 22 percent less likely to get arthritis, compared with those who ate less fish.

The kinds of fish rich in omega-3s include tuna, sardines, salmon, herring, bluefish, mackerel, trout, anchovies, and lake whitefish. If you're not a big fish fan, you can get your omega-3s in fish oil capsules. The most effective dose for relieving arthritis symptoms is between 3 and 5 grams every day, but it may take several weeks before you notice an improvement.

Savor some plant oils. If you have rheumatoid arthritis (RA), replacing some of the fats in your diet with olive oil may help your aching joints. One study found that a Mediterranean diet rich in olive oil reduced production of a substance that causes inflammation in RA.

Some unusual oils may also help reduce joint inflammation in people with RA. These oils include evening primrose, flaxseed, rapeseed, and borage seed oils. They contain a fatty acid similar to omega-3 called gammalinolenic acid (GLA). Because these oils aren't normally found in the foods you eat, you can get them from supplements. The effective dose is 1 to 2 grams daily.

Another recent study found that an unusual combination of plant oils may help the pain of osteoarthritis. Researchers gave an oil extract made from soybeans and avocados, called avocado/soybean unsaponifiables (ASU), or a placebo to people with severe osteoarthritis of the hip or knee. After two months, the ASU group had significantly less pain and disability than the people taking the placebo. No side effects were reported, and the people in the study who took the ASU capsules continued to experience some benefits for about two months after the study was over.

Fill up on veggies. Studies have indicated that a vegetarian diet may lessen the symptoms of rheumatoid arthritis. It isn't clear why vegetarianism seems to be good for arthritis — whether it's a positive effect of the foods you are eating or the foods you aren't eating, like red meat. Scientists think meat affects the types of fatty acids in your blood, which can lead to inflammation.

If you decide to avoid meat, make sure you get enough protein from other sources. Beans, peas, bread, corn, nuts, and wheat germ are good sources of protein.

Munch on some grapes. You've heard that drinking moderate amounts of red wine may be good for your heart. A substance in the skin of grapes used to make the wine — trans-resveratrol — is believed to be responsible for that healthy benefit. Now research indicates that trans-resveratrol may also help reduce the inflammation that contributes to arthritis pain.

A test-tube study found that trans-resveratrol blocked the activation of a gene that contributes to the creation of an enzyme involved in the production of prostaglandins. Prostaglandins are hormone-like substances that can cause inflammation. Although the research is very preliminary and hasn't been tested in humans, you may soon hear that trans-resveratrol can be used to reduce inflammation in people with arthritis.

Because it isn't certain that trans-resveratrol will help relieve arthritis, don't start drinking alcohol, or increase your drinking, especially if you're currently taking pain medication for your arthritis. There's a healthy, harmless way to get some inflammation-fighting trans-resveratrol — eat more grapes.

Spice up your life. If you enjoy spicy Indian food, you might be getting some extra help for the ache of arthritis. Turmeric, the main ingredient in curry, contains a natural antioxidant and anti-inflammatory substance called curcumin. Curcumin gives turmeric its yellow color, and researchers think it may block the release of compounds that cause joint inflammation.

Grab hold of ginger. This spice may work as a natural anti-inflammatory, reducing the swelling and pain of arthritic joints. In one study in Denmark, researchers gave ginger to people with arthritis or muscle pain and found that it relieved muscle discomfort, pain, and swelling in 75 percent of the people. These people took an average of 5 grams of fresh ginger or 1 gram of powdered ginger daily.

Eliminate the offenders. In rheumatoid arthritis, your body's own immune system sends out cells that attack your joints, causing painful inflammation. When you eat a food you are allergic to, your immune system releases cells to fight the offending substance, but those cells could end up attacking your joints instead.

To find out if food allergies are causing your arthritis, try eliminating certain foods from your diet one at a time until you see an improvement. Just remember that arthritis symptoms tend to come and go, and the relief you feel after eliminating a particular food could be a coincidence. Try eating the trouble-making food again to see if it causes symptoms.

The foods most often thought to aggravate arthritis include milk; shrimp; wheat products; certain meats; and nightshade vegetables like tomatoes, potatoes, eggplant, and bell peppers.

Multi-talented vitamins foil arthritis pain

Just as a dose of high-quality plant food can give you luscious, blooming plants, food loaded with nutrients will give you a strong, healthy body. But certain nutrients can do more than just enhance your overall well-being — they can even fight disease and pain. Arthritis is one of those diseases that may respond to vitamins, according to recent medical research.

Folic acid and vitamins B12, C, and D have now become part of the front-line defense against osteoarthritis, a painful condition of the joints that affects more than 50 million people in the United States. Osteoarthritis causes the cartilage in your joints to deteriorate. Your joints no longer move smoothly, and you may feel lots of pain. Luckily, these amazing vitamins can help.

Fend off pain with B vitamins. Researchers in Missouri tested people with osteoarthritis in the joints of their hands. Those who were given a combination of two B vitamins, folic acid (vitamin B9) and cobalamin (vitamin B12), had as much gripping power as people who took NSAIDs (nonsteroidal anti-inflammatory drugs), such as aspirin or ibuprofen. The people taking the vitamin supplements also had fewer tender joints than those who took NSAIDs. Pain did not completely disappear in the people taking the vitamins, but it could easily be controlled with acetaminophen (Tylenol) when necessary.

One big benefit of taking B vitamins for your arthritis is that they don't have the unhealthy side effects NSAIDs have. The people in the study took 6,400 mcg (micrograms) of folic acid and 20 mcg of cobalamin daily.

If you want to try these vitamins to relieve your arthritis pain, ask your doctor to write a prescription. This will enable you to get a large enough dose conveniently and inexpensively.

Safeguard your joints with vitamin C. This well-known vitamin is abundant in many of the foods you eat, such as oranges, strawberries, cantaloupe, sweet red peppers, tomatoes, brussels sprouts, and collard greens. It's also a common supplement available in every pharmacy and most discount and grocery stores.

Vitamin C is important because of its antioxidant properties — it naturally fights disease and damage in many parts of your body. According to a recent study at the Boston University Medical Center, one of the areas it helps is the cartilage in your knees.

A group of 640 people were tested to see if a high intake of vitamin C would help prevent cartilage loss and osteoarthritis of the knee joints. In the people who consumed the least vitamin C, the disease progressed three times faster than in those with the highest intake.

For the people who took in lots of vitamin C, there was also less knee pain. Considering the benefits, there is nothing to lose and everything to gain by increasing your intake of vitamin C. Some experts recommend getting at least twice the recommended dietary allowance (RDA) of 75 milligrams (mg) for women and 90 mg for men. One cup of fresh orange juice has about 120 mg.

Although natural food sources are best, it's generally safe to take a supplement if you need to.

Fortify your cartilage with vitamin D. Here's where vitamin D comes in. Calcium makes up the basic building blocks of your bones, but it takes vitamin D to make your body absorb it. Doctors who recently researched the role of vitamin D in osteoarthritis think the cartilage in your joints may be protected by the vitamin. They think it's also possible vitamin D may actually keep the bones of the joints intact. No matter how it works — the results are clear. If you have osteoarthritis, make sure you're getting enough vitamin D. If your intake is low, the risk of your arthritis getting worse is three times as great.

The best source of this valuable nutrient is simple sunshine. When you're exposed to sunlight, your body manufactures vitamin D. If you get out in the sun for about 30 minutes every day, you'll get all you need. You can also get vitamin D in fortified milk; boiled shrimp; eggs; and fatty fish, such as salmon, tuna, and sardines. Only take vitamin D supplements under your doctor's care — too much can be toxic. If you live in a climate that is more cloudy than sunny, or you can't get outside much, this might be a good option for you.

Now that you know what folic acid and vitamins B12, C, and D can do for osteoarthritis, there's no reason why you shouldn't take advantage of these powerful nutrients to help keep joint pain and stiffness in check.

Tackle arthritis with these 10 tips

Much of life involves learning to cope with challenges and finding out which strategies work for you and which don't. If you have arthritis, here are some ways you can adapt your surroundings to make your challenges easier to meet:

▶ To make a pen or pencil easier to grasp, have someone twist a large rubber band around it just below the area where your fingers rest. Or take the plastic center out of a foam hair roller and slide a pencil into the center of the foam. You can also get a pencil grip made of soft rubber where school supplies are sold. A ballpoint pen is easier to use than a felt-tip pen or pencil.

▶ Ask someone to help you raise your bed. You won't have to bend over when you make it. Using knitted sheets that stretch will also help you make your bed with ease.

▶ To help you tuck in your sheets and blankets, use a wooden pizza paddle.

▶ Consider buying a speakerphone to replace your regular telephone so you don't get a stiff or sore neck and shoulder from cradling the receiver for long periods of time.

▶ When you're reading, place the book on several pillows in your lap to raise it to a comfortable height. To turn the pages of a book, use the eraser end of a pencil or a rubber fingertip. Blow gently along the edges to separate the pages.

▶ To play a game of cards without aching hands, insert the cards into the side of a closed box of aluminum foil or waxed paper. You can also put the bottom of a shoe box into its lid and stand cards in the space between the box and the lid.

▶ In the kitchen, create a lower work space so you can sit while working. Pull out a drawer and place a cookie sheet over the opening. Roll jars and bottles on the counter instead of shaking them. Open a bottle or jar more easily by having someone wind a rubber band around the lid.

▶ If you have trouble gripping your car door handle, especially when it's cold or wet, glue a piece of rubber (like the kind that opens jars) to the underside of the door handle. Make your steering wheel easier to grip by padding it with a foam cover (available in automotive stores). And add extra cushioning to the car seat to keep your back, hips, and legs more comfortable while driving.

▶ If you have trouble standing up for a shower, try putting a webbed lawn chair in the shower stall so you can sit while you bathe. It's easier to dry off after a shower by putting on a terry cloth bathrobe. And if you're bathing a baby in a sink or bathtub, wear a soft cotton glove on the supporting hand to keep him from slipping out of your grasp.

▶ When you're getting dressed, put the garment on your weaker limb first. When undressing, take the garment off the stronger limb first. Try knee-high or thigh-high hose to eliminate the hassle of putting on pantyhose.

Set your aching joints free with tai chi

Years ago, doctors didn't advise people with arthritis to exercise. They thought that too much activity would cause the arthritis to get worse. But studies now show that if you don't use your muscles, they'll lose their strength, and the joints you don't move will just get stiffer.

Exercise can reduce the amount of medication needed to control pain and increase strength and flexibility. It may even delay or prevent arthritis from developing in other joints. Yet the wrong kind of exercise can damage your joints even further and make your arthritis worse. So what's a person to do?

Perhaps it's time to try a different kind of exercise — tai chi. This "soft" martial art (unlike karate, with aggressive kicks and punches) has been compared to dancing because of its slow, gently rhythmic movements, one flowing into another. And the steps are always practiced in the same order — like a choreographed dance. That makes it quick to learn and easy to remember.

Best of all, tai chi has been proven helpful to people with arthritis. It's an exercise that involves the major joints of the body and is good for people of any age. You can do it at your own pace and start seeing results right away.

Just ask Dr. Paul Lam, a family physician in Sydney, Australia. He took up the practice of tai chi more than 20 years ago when he found himself with symptoms of arthritis. He got his arthritis under control and went on to enter tai chi competitions, even winning a gold medal.

As he taught others to do tai chi over the years, Dr. Lam adapted the traditional forms to make it easier for people with health problems. Eventually, he developed a 12-movement program specifically for arthritis sufferers. His *Tai Chi for Arthritis* program is endorsed as a safe and therapeutic tool by the Arthritis Foundation of Australia.

"We have many groups," says Dr. Lam, "and approximately 90 percent report significant improvement within weeks. I get mail regularly from my 'video' students telling me of amazing results."

With practice, tai chi improves your flexibility and the range of movement of your joints. It also strengthens and tones your muscles. Dr. Lam thinks that's particularly important because strong muscles protect your joints.

And for those who take up tai chi early in life, they may help themselves avoid the pain of arthritis later on. Although there's no proof of this just yet, Dr. Lam is optimistic. "We do believe tai chi helps to prevent development of at least osteoarthritis. There is indirect evidence for it."

If you're interested in trying out this gentle martial art, check with your local hospital, health and fitness club, or community recreation department to see if they offer classes. If you prefer the comfort of your home, you can order Dr. Lam's *Tai Chi for Arthritis* videotape through his website <www.taichiproductions.com> or purchase it through a major bookstore like Borders.

Here are some suggestions for making the most of your tai chi program:

▶ Before you start, talk to your doctor. He can advise you about the level of activity you are ready to handle.

▶ Look for a teacher who will take time to plan with you and help you develop at your own pace.

▶ Encourage a friend or your spouse to try it with you. Teaming up with a companion or a group will make it even more enjoyable as you support each other's efforts.

▶ If you have foot pain, wear well-cushioned athletic shoes and try to distribute your weight evenly as you move through the various forms.

▶ Listen to your body. If a particular posture or movement is painful, make adjustments. If you get tired, stop and rest. There is no need to push yourself.

While you're increasing your strength, flexibility, and endurance, you may be surprised to find you feel more relaxed as well. According to Dr. Lam, tai chi has the added benefit of relieving the anxiety and depression that sometimes accompany arthritis.

"When people begin to improve and to restore their lifestyle, dignity, and freedom, they gain confidence to overcome their anxiety and depression. Exercise," he affirms, "gives people an uplifting in spirit."

2 'hot' supplements you need to know about

If you suffer from joint pain, you've probably been tempted to try a dietary supplement. Beware — some supplements have research to confirm their effectiveness, while others are still unproven. Here's the scoop on two of the most popular supplements for joint health.

Loosen up with glucosamine. You may have heard of this "hot" new supplement for the treatment of arthritis. Actually, glucosamine has been used for decades to treat arthritis in horses and dogs, and it's been available for human use in Europe since the 1980s. But in the

United States, it only became popular after publication of the book *The Arthritis Cure* (St. Martin's Press, 1997) by Jason Theodosakis, a medical doctor and lecturer in preventative medicine.

Glucosamine is a natural compound of glucose and amino acids. It forms the main ingredient for most of the connective and cushioning tissue in your body. It is the breakdown of these tissues — such as cartilage and synovial fluids — that causes the pain and immobility of arthritis.

The theory behind glucosamine supplements is that if you replace this important building block, your joint tissue will start to build up again. And several studies have found evidence that the theory just might work.

In fact, glucosamine may be at least as effective as NSAIDs in controlling the pain and stiffness of osteoarthritis, but it may take longer to feel the effect. In one study, people with arthritis were given either ibuprofen or glucosamine. The people taking ibuprofen reported more pain relief in the first and second weeks than the people taking glucosamine, but by the fourth week, both groups had about the same level of pain relief. By the eighth week, glucosamine was slightly more effective than ibuprofen. Glucosamine also caused fewer side effects, like stomach discomfort, than ibuprofen.

You can buy several forms of glucosamine supplements. The most common, and probably most effective, is glucosamine sulfate. The recommended dosage, according to results from studies, is 1,500 milligrams (mg) a day, taken in three doses of 500 mg each.

Get the facts about MSM. Another "hot" supplement being used to treat arthritis symptoms is methylsulfonylmethane (MSM). It is chemically related to DMSO (dimethyl sulfoxide), which was a "hot" new supplement 20 years ago.

Both MSM and DMSO contain sulfur, which your body needs to form disulfide bonds. These bonds hold together body tissues like hair, skin, nails, and joints. You can get sulfur from your diet. It is found in meats, fish, eggs, milk, legumes, nuts, garlic, and poultry.

Because sulfur is important to your body's tissues, including the cartilage needed to cushion your joints, it is possible that MSM may help relieve arthritis symptoms. But research on MSM supplements for joint pain is skimpy, with no major studies to confirm its effectiveness.

Still, manufacturers of MSM claim it relieves stress, asthma, arthritis, inflammation, constipation, muscle cramps, and back pain and increases blood circulation, energy, alertness, mental calmness, and the ability to concentrate. Usually, claims that any one supplement is the solution to so many different conditions is a red flag that you shouldn't waste your money. Nevertheless, many people are buying MSM and believe it works for them. So far, no side effects have been reported.

Soothe achy joints with natural healers

Wouldn't you like to find a natural alternative to over-the-counter pain relievers for the ache of arthritis? A sweet-smelling flower and a red-hot pepper may provide natural relief.

Cool the pain with capsaicin's heat. Research has found that capsaicin, the active ingredient in red peppers, is effective in relieving arthritis pain. But you don't have to grow the peppers in your garden. Ready-made relief is available at your nearest drugstore in an over-the-counter cream. Made from dried cayenne peppers, capsaicin cream is absorbed through your skin and works by deadening local nerves.

Using capsaicin can make exercise less painful and enable you to follow a regular exercise schedule. If you have osteoarthritis, exercise helps relieve pain, increase mobility, and prevent muscle loss.

Even if capsaicin doesn't totally relieve your arthritis pain, it may help reduce the amount of other drugs you take. It is applied directly to your skin, which means it shouldn't interact with any medication you take by mouth.

Capsaicin doesn't seem to have any adverse side effects, even after prolonged use. It appears to be as safe and effective now as it was centuries ago when the Mayan and Incan Indians used it to treat arthritis.

Soak up arnica's gentle relief. These beautiful yellow and orange flowers have been used for centuries as a safe and effective external treatment. Arnica's healing benefits include relieving pain from bruises, sprains, and aches; easing hemorrhoid pain; helping heal scrapes and cuts; stopping the itch from insect bites; and easing the ache of arthritis.

Arnica speeds healing partly because it has a natural antibiotic effect, and partly because it increases circulation in small blood vessels. According to researchers, using arnica compresses on arthritic joints brings relief from soreness and stiffness because it acts like a painkiller.

To make an arnica compress, dilute a tablespoon of arnica tincture in two cups of water. Soak gauze pads or other absorbent material and apply to the affected area.

You can buy arnica tincture at health food stores or pharmacies that sell natural and homeopathic medicines.

A word of caution — arnica is for external use only. If taken internally, it is poisonous, causing elevated blood pressure and cardiac arrest. Also, some people are sensitive to an ingredient in arnica and may develop a rash from using the compress.

Although these two remedies may not totally relieve your arthritis pain, they may offer some relief without the side effects of most oral medication.

Emergency aid for aches and pains

Acute attacks of arthritis pain require rest. Many doctors and physical therapists will let you decide whether heat or ice makes your painful joints feel better. Give your body a break, and take the time to pamper it with a homemade heating pad or ice pack. Say goodbye to muscle aches and arthritis pain, and say hello to these free fast remedies.

Turn up the heat. Warmth relaxes sore muscles, stimulates blood circulation, and eases stiff joints on a chilly day. Avoid combining heat therapy with pain-killing cream, or you could end up with severe burns.

▶ Dampen a hand towel or washcloth and zap it in the microwave until it's warm and steamy. Just be careful not to overheat it.

▶ Baby your joints with a hot water bottle, and place a towel between it and your skin.

▶ Fill an old clean sock with rice or salt, and tie or sew the end closed. Heat it in the microwave until warm, but not hot, then lay it on your aching joint.

▶ Wet the pad of a disposable diaper and pop it in the microwave. Let it cool down if you overheat it, then wrap this unusual heating pad around your sore spots.

Chill out. Cold relieves pain by numbing pain-sensing nerves and reducing inflammation.

▶ Make a slushy ice pack to mold around any injury. Mix one part rubbing alcohol with three parts water in a zip-lock bag. The alcohol will keep it from freezing completely, resulting in frozen "slush." Wrap it in a cloth and apply to the injury.

▶ Place unpopped popcorn kernels into a zip-lock freezer bag and keep in the freezer.

▶ Fill an uninflated balloon or a disposable rubber glove with water and freeze.

▶ Wet a clean sock, stick it in a zip-lock bag, and freeze.

Don't be fooled by arthritis impostors

Achy, swollen joints usually indicate arthritis, but sometimes joint pain can be triggered by these temporary and reversible conditions.

Human parvovirus B19. This virus can trigger prolonged arthritis pain. Other symptoms include a flu-like illness with fever, headache, muscle aches, and sometimes nausea and vomiting. Many times these first symptoms are followed by the appearance of a rash, although the rash is much more common in children than in adults. The arthritis symptoms caused by parvovirus usually go away within a month, but some people will suffer with joint pain for several months.

The people most likely to get parvovirus B19 are those with weakened immune systems, like people with AIDS, chronic anemia, or sickle cell anemia. Scientists are working on a vaccine to help prevent complications in people at high risk.

Food poisoning. Your aching joints may be a result of the same thing that caused your stomachache, nausea, and diarrhea a few weeks ago. Sometimes *Salmonella* bacteria, which cause a type of food poisoning, can also cause reactive arthritis a few weeks after infection.

The most common source of *Salmonella* is raw eggs, but it can also be found in raw meats, poultry, milk and dairy products, fish, shrimp, salad dressing, cake mixes, cream-filled desserts, peanut butter, and chocolate. To protect yourself, never eat anything that contains raw eggs, and cook all meats thoroughly. If you order a dish in a restaurant that could contain raw or undercooked eggs, such as Hollandaise sauce or Caesar salad dressing, make sure the restaurant uses pasteurized eggs.

Drug side effects. Some prescription drugs cause joint pain as a side effect. If you think your medicine may be causing your pain, ask your doctor. Don't stop taking the medication without your doctor's advice.

Here's a partial list of drugs that can cause painful joints.

Generic drug name	Common brand names	Conditions drug treats
acyclovir	Zovirax	viruses, especially herpes zoster (shingles)
amiloride	Midamor, Moduretic	high blood pressure, congestive heart failure
carbamazepine	Carbatrol, Tegretol	seizures
doxycycline	Doryx, Vibramycin	infections
famotidine	Pepcid, Mylanta AR	ulcers
hydrochlorothiazide	Aldoril, Dyazide, Inderide, Lopressor	high blood pressure
hydroflumethiazide	Diucardin	congestive heart failure
isotretinoin	Accutane	acne
lovastatin	Mevacor	high cholesterol
methylphenidate	Ritalin	attention deficit disorder, narcolepsy

mexiletine	Mexitil	irregular heartbeat
minocycline	Dynacin, Minocin, Vectrin	infections
neostigmine	Prostigmin	myasthenia gravis
nicotine	Habitrol, Nicoderm, Nicotrol, Prostep	cigarette addiction
nifedipine	Adalat, Procardia	angina
paroxetine	Paxil	depression
pergolide	Permax	Parkinson's disease
sulfamethoxazole	Bactrim, Septra	infections
verapamil	Calan, Covera-HS, Isoptin SR, Verelan	angina, irregular heartbeat, high blood pressure

Sweet substitute relieves pain

If you drink diet sodas or use a sugar substitute in your coffee, you may help ease your arthritis pain. Research finds that the popular artificial sweetener aspartame may serve as an effective substitute for certain pain relievers.

Allen Edmundson, a researcher at the Oklahoma Medical Research Foundation, suspected that the aspartame in his diet cola was responsible for lowering his arthritis pain. He tested his theory and found that people with osteoarthritis who took aspartame could walk farther with less pain, climb stairs faster, and grip things more easily.

Another study found that aspartame was as effective as non-steroidal anti-inflammatory drugs (NSAIDs) in reducing fever in laboratory rats.

Although these are small, preliminary studies, researchers are encouraged by the results because many people who take NSAIDs suffer from serious side effects. Most people should have no side effects from aspartame if they take in the small amounts found in a half or full can of diet soda.

Some people maintain that aspartame can cause health problems or worsen certain conditions such as lupus and fibromyalgia. There is no scientific evidence to support that, but if you have concerns about using aspartame, be sure and talk to your health care provider.

Asthma

Breathe deeper for asthma relief

During your lifetime you may take more than a hundred million breaths. And chances are you won't pay attention to most of them, unless you have a respiratory problem — like asthma. In that case, you'll notice the wheezing and the frightening feeling that comes when you can't get enough air.

But you can breathe easier with asthma if you learn to breathe better. A group of 4,741 people with asthma were asked in a survey about alternative treatments they had tried. The most common response was breathing techniques, especially from those with severe asthma. And most of the asthma sufferers said they found the exercises helpful.

Scientific studies show you can improve the functioning of your lungs and reduce your need for medication by learning to breathe better. You can also improve your mental outlook and spend more time being physically active.

Psychologist and breathing expert Dr. Gay Hendricks has taught "conscious breathing" to many people with asthma. To learn his technique, read *Banish stress with better breathing* in the *Stress* chapter, but check with your doctor before you begin. For people with asthma, he offers these additional suggestions.

Make a lifetime commitment. "Asthma can feel like a frightening and complex problem, but the solutions are often quite simple," says Hendricks. He finds that training people to breathe deeply is the quickest way to get the most benefit. Then, as you get results, he encourages you to think of conscious breathing as a lifelong practice.

Let it all out. Hendricks says most people with asthma don't empty their lungs when they breathe out. "They tend to hold air in," he says, "particularly high in their chests."

He believes this is probably an emotional response to the fear that if you completely let go of a breath, you may not get another good one. But with practice, you can learn to feel comfortable about pushing all the air out. You'll know there will be another, as Hendricks puts it, "free for the taking."

Drink lots of water. "Keeping moist is important," says Hendricks, "especially in climates where the air is very dry. But even if you live in a humid climate, extra breathing can dry out the sensitive passages of your airways." Keep a glass of water nearby and drink often when you are practicing conscious breathing.

Stop if you feel dizzy. While you are doing the breathing exercises, your body is adjusting to getting more oxygen. You may experience dizziness or some other unusual sensation. This could mean you are trying too hard. "Rest until it has passed," says Hendricks, "or return to the activities on another occasion. Better to take them slow and easy."

Be patient with yourself. Dr. Hendricks says deep breathing exercises can require a lot of effort for people with asthma. Since frustration can trigger an asthma attack, it's important to remain calm.

Practice for a few minutes, then rest. Having a helper with you while you practice may make it easier. If impatience interferes with the exercises, you might want to work with a psychologist, like Hendricks, or other professional breathing coach.

For specific breathing exercises designed especially for people with asthma, check out Hendricks' book, *Conscious Breathing*, published by Bantam Books. You may find it at your local library or bookstore. Or you can order it, and his audio and videotapes as well, from his website <www.hendricks.com>.

3 natural 'prescriptions' for asthma relief

It's easy to take breathing for granted, but if you have asthma, breathing doesn't always come easy. For natural relief, consider the herb ginkgo, the spice turmeric, or magnesium — a vital mineral.

Breathe comfortably with ginkgo. For more than a millennium, people in Asia have looked to the ginkgo tree as a source of healing. In recent years, scientists have discovered how ginkgo can make breathing more comfortable for people with asthma.

The same substance that causes your blood to clot when you get a cut can trigger an asthma attack. It's called PAF or platelet activating factor. PAF can cause allergic responses, including bronchospasms. This sudden narrowing of the main air passages from the windpipe to the lungs may feel like a tightening or squeezing in your chest, and breathing becomes difficult. Ginkgo can prevent this by blocking PAF.

Ginkgo biloba extract, sometimes called GBE or GBX, is sold as an herbal supplement in health food stores. You can get it in liquid form or as tablets or capsules.

The extract should be 24 percent flavoglycosides, 10 percent of which should be quercetin. It should also contain 6 percent terpenoids. Look on the label for the words "tannin-free" and "50:1 concentrate." The 50:1 ratio means it took 50 pounds of leaves to produce 1 pound of extract.

The recommended dosage is 40 milligrams (mg) taken three times a day. You may have to take the supplement for four to six weeks before you notice any effects.

No serious side effects have been reported, but some people experience headaches or mild digestive problems.

Tame wheezing with turmeric. The plant curcuma longa grows wild in Java, but you probably have some of the spice that comes from its tuber-like rhizomes in your pantry.

The spice is turmeric, a main ingredient of curry powder. It's the pigment in turmeric, called curcumin, that gives curry its yellow color. This pigment, according to researchers from the Nihon University School of Medicine in Tokyo, can also help prevent asthma attacks. The curcumin curbs the release of substances that cause the symptoms of asthma, like wheezing and chest-tightening.

Although the study didn't specify a certain amount, the usual dose of turmeric for other conditions is 1.5 to 3 grams daily. You can get supplements in capsule or liquid form at health food stores. There are no known side effects from turmeric except occasional stomach upsets after prolonged use. If you have gallstones or a blockage of the bile duct, you shouldn't use it.

Stop muscle spasms with magnesium. Avocado, sunflower seeds, and pinto beans contain a lot of magnesium, which may help your lungs fight the muscle spasms of asthma attacks. In fact, doctors sometimes treat asthma with magnesium sulfate.

The recommended dietary allowance (RDA) for magnesium is 320 mg for women over 30 and 420 mg for men over 30. Supplements are available, but your body can absorb the mineral better if you get it naturally from food. Nuts, legumes, seafood, and dark green vegetables are good sources of magnesium. Since it is easily lost during washing, peeling, and processing, choose fresh or minimally processed foods.

When it comes to magnesium, moderation is the key word. Too much can make you very sick, causing nausea, vomiting, or even paralysis or death. Getting too much magnesium from the foods you eat is usually not a problem. But magnesium is a main ingredient in some over-the-counter medication, including laxatives and antacids.

If you regularly consume large amounts of these drugs, you may be poisoning yourself. Check the label on any medication you are taking.

A nippy dip stops asthma cold

Just the thought of stepping into a cold bath may take your breath away. But if you are bothered by the wheezing and chest-squeezing feelings of asthma attacks, you can take comfort from an icy dip.

Research shows cold water baths can improve breathing — but don't stay in there too long. A quick bath in cold water for only one minute or a 30-second cold shower every day showed the greatest results.

So turn on the cold water, brace yourself, and jump in — and enjoy easy breathing.

Athlete's Foot

How to give athlete's foot the boot

Athlete's foot really has nothing to do with sports, other than its reputation for being passed around locker rooms. Actually, the condition is caused by a fungus everyone has growing on their skin.

The fungus thrives on warmth and moisture, which is why it loves sweaty feet. If you wear tight shoes and socks, especially in a warm climate, or don't dry your feet promptly and completely after bathing, you're the perfect target for an athlete's foot attack.

This common skin condition can cause a simple redness and rash on the bottom and sides of your feet or blisters and cracked and peeling skin between your toes. In some cases, toenail infections occur that can cause splitting or loss of the nail.

It is not known why some people develop athlete's foot and some don't. What is known is what you can do to prevent it.

▶ Wash your feet every day and dry them completely, paying special attention to the skin between your toes.

▶ Don't wear tight shoes and heavy socks. Sandals are great but going barefoot is even better.

▶ When you wear shoes, choose socks made from a natural fiber, like cotton. The cotton will draw moisture away from your skin. If your socks get sweaty, change them as soon as you can.

▶ Every now and then, sprinkle some anti-fungal powder into your shoes. It helps keep them dry and will attack any fungus that may be lurking, waiting to climb onto your feet.

▶ If you spend time in locker rooms or other such places, don't go in there with bare feet. Get yourself some shower shoes or flip-flops. Although athlete's foot is not as contagious as most people believe, community showers and bathrooms are still no place for bare feet. The constant warmth and moisture, plus the heavy traffic, combine to create the perfect breeding ground for foot fungus.

The good news about this itchy pest is that it's easily treated with an over-the-counter anti-fungal cream. But before you go self-medicating, even with creams, make sure the rash on your foot is athlete's foot. Not all rashes are caused by athlete's foot, and using the wrong medication on a rash can make the problem worse.

In more severe cases, ask your doctor for help. He can prescribe foot soaks or oral medication. To prevent the infection from coming back, don't stop using the cream or medication as soon as the rash disappears and the itching stops. Those signs alone don't mean the fungus is gone.

These two tips might also help prevent future attacks.

▶ Toss out any shoes you wore without socks while you had the fungus. This might seem like an expensive way to prevent reinfection, but consider it an investment in your foot's health. If the fungus is alive in those shoes, they can just keep giving it to you over and over again.

▶ Every once in a while, rub some anti-fungal cream between your toes, over your nails, and on the bottoms of your feet. This will keep any lingering or new fungi from getting ideas on settling in the neighborhood.

Back Pain

7 ways to escape back pain

Most people take their backs for granted until something goes wrong. Don't wait to become one of the 80 percent of people affected by back problems. Start babying your back today to avoid back problems tomorrow.

Watch out for bad posture. Practice good posture at all times — keep your back straight, not arched, and your shoulders level. Don't slump even when you're relaxing. If you have to stand for long periods, rest one foot on a low stool and shift your weight often. Wear comfortable shoes with good support and low heels. Change positions frequently, no matter what you're doing.

Sit up straight. Choose a chair that gives your lower back good support. Add a small cushion or rolled-up towel to the small of your back, even when you're driving. Sit properly with both feet on the floor or on a low stool, and keep your hips and legs at a 90-degree angle. Keep your chair close enough to your desk so you don't have to lean forward. If you spend a lot of time sitting, get up now and then to stretch.

Practice safe lifting. Keep your spine straight. Either squat, bending your knees, or bend at the hips — not the waist. Use your arms and legs to lift and keep the object close to your body.

Enjoy restful sleep. If you sleep on your back, put a pillow under your knees. If you sleep on your side, keep your knees bent.

Get some exercise. A simple exercise program, combining aerobic, flexibility, and strengthening exercises, will help keep your back in good shape. Try to exercise for at least 30 minutes every other day. And remember to check with your doctor before starting an exercise program.

Stop smoking. Smoking has been linked to many back disorders. Researchers say smoking makes bones weaker by slowing the production of new bone cells. Weak bones can cause back pain.

Maintain a healthy weight. If you're overweight, lose those extra pounds. They are putting even more pressure on your spine.

Conquer back pain with no-sweat workout

The best way to prevent back pain and injury is to strengthen the muscles that surround and support your spine. Here are four exercises that will help you steer clear of back pain. Do your back workout at least three days a week, beginning with two or three repetitions and working up to 10 for each exercise.

Lie on the floor with your knees bent and your feet flat. Suck in your stomach muscles and lift your seat off the floor. Starting at your shoulders, relax your back and slowly flatten it against the floor. Hold your back flat against the floor for a count of five and then relax.

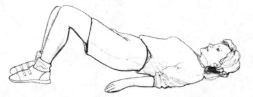

Beginning in the same position, fold your arms across your chest. Lift your head and shoulders slowly off the floor to a 45-degree angle, trying to feel the pull in your stomach muscles, not your neck. Hold for a count of five, then relax.

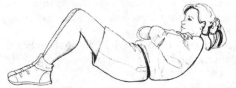

Lie flat on your back with both legs out straight. Grab one knee and pull it straight back toward your chest. Point your foot toward your head. Hold for a count of five, then repeat with the other leg.

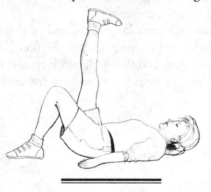

Lie flat on your back with both knees bent. Lift one leg toward the ceiling with your knee straight and your foot pointed toward your head. Stretch your leg as far as possible over your head, holding for a count of five. Relax, and repeat with the other leg.

Don't take back pain lightly

Many times an aching back is simply a warning to change the way you sit, stand, and lift — a wake-up call that things could get worse. But sometimes back pain is a sign of a serious problem.

If your back pain was caused by a fall or injury or it's accompanied by weak or numb legs, fever, or shooting pain below your knee, see your doctor right away.

Back pain that's not relieved by several weeks of self-treatment is another good reason to seek professional help.

Chronic back pain could be a symptom of any of these serious conditions:

- a kidney infection or stone
- reproductive problems in women
- prostate problems in men

- cancer of the spine, intestines, or pancreas
- scoliosis (curvature of the spine)

Don't hesitate to see a specialist if your family doctor has trouble diagnosing the cause of your pain.

---

3 tips to soothe an aching back

Back pain is often a sign of a serious condition, but if you're sure you don't have a medical problem that needs professional attention, your discomfort is probably from overdoing it.

First of all, stop doing whatever caused the attack. Don't try to work through the pain. Being tough won't win you any trophies. Then try these pain-relieving tips, and you'll be back in the swing of things before you know it.

Grab a pill and a pillow. Taking aspirin or ibuprofen is a quick way to stop the pain. These over-the-counter painkillers not only attack the discomfort, they also have anti-inflammatory power to help shrink swollen, inflamed muscles. Relax by lying on your back with a pillow under your knees or on your side with a pillow between your knees.

Cool it or warm it. An ice pack and a gentle back massage may help cool your searing pain. Here's a simple kitchen remedy that will combine the two. Fill a small paper cup with water and freeze it solid. Have your spouse or a friend tear the paper off one end of the cup, then use the ice to massage your aching muscles. Try to hang in there for about 10 minutes, repeating as often as once an hour. If heat soothes you better, treat your back to a warm heating pad. Just be sure to turn it off before you fall asleep.

Get some rest — then get going. A day of bed rest may be needed and deserved when your back is really hurting, but don't overstay your welcome. A recent study showed that back-pain sufferers who went about their daily activities got well faster than those who exercised or stayed in bed. Get up as soon as you feel like it, even for short periods. Resume your normal activities, but take things easy for a

while. Save that tennis match for later when your body can bounce
back as easily as the ball.

Give yourself a back-soothing massage

Can't quite fit a masseuse into your weekly budget? Try this
easy at-home way to give yourself a back-pleasing massage.

Put four tennis balls inside a long sock. Lie down so your
lower back is resting on the sock. Roll gently up and down and
side to side. Your body weight will place just enough pressure on
the tennis balls to give your muscles a good rubdown.

Look before you leap into back surgery

Your back pain started a few weeks ago. You try to rest and take
it easy, but the pain just won't go away. Finally, you make a trip to the
doctor and a magnetic resonance imaging (MRI) scan shows that you
have a ruptured disk. Your doctor says you may need surgery.

Wait! Before you panic and undergo risky back surgery, you need
to know the facts. Not all ruptured disks cause pain and problems. A
recent study of 98 people with no back pain revealed that over half of
them had one or more ruptured disks. Since a damaged disk does not
necessarily hurt, it might be a coincidence that you have a sore back
and a ruptured disk.

Disks are the soft, rounded cartilage between the bones of the
spine. A ruptured disk occurs if the jelly-like interior of the disk is
pushed out of its usual place and extends beyond the bones of the
spine. Ruptured disks are also called herniated, protruding, or slipped
disks. Often, ruptured disks shrink over time, returning to fit their
normal spaces again.

Most people with back pain improve without surgery. In fact, the
long-term results of people who have surgery are identical to those
who don't. Consider the results of another study of 126 people with
ruptured disks. Half the group underwent surgery. The other half

were treated without surgery. Four years later, the two groups showed very little, if any, difference.

Usually doctors don't know why your back hurts. Doctors aren't able to identify a definite cause of pain in 85 percent of the people who come to them with back complaints. In addition, the number of surgeries on the lumbar spine, or lower back, increases with the growth of new imaging techniques, such as MRI. When an MRI reveals a ruptured disk, doctors are likely to point to that as the cause of your back pain. The cure they will probably suggest — surgery.

But interpretations of an MRI scan can vary from doctor to doctor. If your doctor suggests back surgery based on the results of imaging testing, get a second opinion. Keep in mind that 96 percent of all back injuries will heal with rest and rehabilitative exercises.

Bad Breath

How to overcome bad breath

Almost everyone has suffered from bad breath from time to time. When you eat, pieces of food get caught between your teeth and on your tongue. They break down and give off foul-smelling gases like hydrogen sulphide.

Although bad breath can be embarrassing, it's easy to fix. These tips should help freshen your breath. If they don't, your bad breath may be a sign of illness you shouldn't ignore.

Keep your mouth clean. Brush your teeth with a soft toothbrush and fluoride toothpaste at least twice a day. Brush well along the gumline and over all tooth surfaces. To remove food and plaque from between your teeth, floss every day. Curve the floss around each tooth to cover the side surfaces.

Don't forget to clean your tongue. It's a huge source of bacteria and odor. If brushing your tongue is uncomfortable, use a special tongue scraper or the side of a spoon to gently scrape that sticky, germy film off your tongue. Either way, be gentle.

Dentures are a common source of bacteria and bad breath. If you have removable dentures, braces, or plates, keep them squeaky clean. Remove and brush them each night, and soak them in a disinfectant solution. Your dentist can tell you the best kind to use.

Beware of mouthwash. Antiseptic and deodorant mouthwashes and sprays only cover up breath odor temporarily — for about 10 minutes to an hour at most.

Mouthwashes containing alcohol can throw off your mouth's natural chemical balance and dry it out, which can cause bad breath. Swish and gargle only if your dentist recommends it.

These homemade mouthwashes may improve your breath without drying out your mouth:

► Mix some Listerine or Cepacol and olive oil. Gargle and spit out three times a day.

► Rinse with a mixture of half hydrogen peroxide and half water (don't gargle).

Prescription mouthwashes containing chlorhexidine seem to be effective in preventing gum disease. In studies, this germ-killing mouth rinse reduced bacteria by 50 percent. If you aren't able to brush and floss properly because of a physical disability, this rinse may help you avoid dental problems.

See your dentist. Get regular dental exams and talk to your dentist about any problems you're having, like ill-fitting crowns. Twice-yearly checkups and cleanings will keep your mouth healthy and sweet-smelling. If you have tooth decay or gum disease, both causes of bad breath, your dentist can fix the problem.

Shy away from certain foods. A spicy lunch, such as garlic chicken, liver and onions, fish, or a pastrami sandwich, can give you "death breath" by afternoon. But did you know eating meat makes your breath more pungent than eating fruits and vegetables? Once the chemical compounds in certain foods get into your bloodstream, your lungs excrete the odor. Breath sprays or mints won't cover it up. Alcohol, coffee, and tobacco (either smoked or chewed) are also causes of bad breath.

Serve up nutritious meals. Eat lots of fresh fruits, vegetables, and whole grains, rather than foods loaded with sugar and fat.

And don't forget calcium — it helps build strong teeth. Skim milk and other low-fat dairy products are good sources. Broccoli, cabbage, cauliflower, beans, and nuts are also high in calcium.

Eating yogurt or drinking buttermilk that contains active cultures will also douse bad breath. The active lactobacillus bacteria make it hard for other odor-causing bacteria to grow.

You can halt "hunger breath" by not skipping meals. If you skip meals, diet, or fast, you aren't supplying your body with enough nutrients, and it will begin to break down your internal supply of protein for energy. This process creates an odor you exhale from your lungs.

Drink lots of water. Saliva constantly washes anything out of your mouth that can cause bad breath. As you get older, your salivary glands produce less saliva. If your mouth is too dry, it generally gives off a bad odor.

Make sure you drink lots of water, at least six to eight glasses a day, but don't constantly rinse your mouth. You may be washing away any saliva that will help fight bad breath.

Suck on hard candies, especially lemon drops. Eat lots of oranges, grapefruit, and other citrus fruits. To stimulate the flow of saliva naturally, eat high-fiber foods, like celery, and chew sugarless gum or parsley.

Dry mouth can also be caused by sinus or throat infections, exercise, stress, mouth-breathing, talking, and certain medications, such as antihistamines, antidepressants, and anticoagulants.

Banish bad breath with green tea

Green tea's pleasant taste and aroma, its low cost, and its role in Eastern traditions have made it a staple in the Far East for more than 2,000 years. But now, modern science is proving that tea has a much more tangible, medicinal value. Available just about anywhere, green tea is more than just a good drink — it's a drink that's good for you.

Research shows that green tea may help fight cancer, heart disease, liver disease, diabetes, and colds and flu. Green tea can also keep your mouth healthy by curbing the growth of bacteria that cause cavities, plaque, and bad breath. What more could you ask from a tiny leaf?

If you can't imagine giving up your familiar bag of black tea, consider this. Green tea is green and black tea is black only because of the way they are processed. The leaves come from the same plant. To make green tea, the leaves are merely picked and steamed — almost no processing at all, which many people believe makes it healthier. To get black tea, the leaves must be processed a lot longer and allowed to ferment. An in-between tea, called Oolong, is still fermented but for less time than black tea.

To make the best cup of green tea, don't allow your water to come to a complete boil — that makes it too hot. Steep the leaves for only about two to three minutes. For some tea drinkers, that may still be too long. Experiment to find out what tea strength suits your taste. You can even use green tea leaves more than once.

As the Japanese would say, "May you live 10,000 years!"

Drugs that cause bad breath

Bad breath can be a side effect of several commonly used drugs. If you are taking one of these, don't stop without your doctor's permission. But if bad breath is really bothering you or your family, ask if there's an alternative.

- Antineoplastic drugs, used to fight cancer, may cause mouth ulcers, bleeding of your gums, or a fungus infection in your mouth.
- Dimethyl sulfoxide (DMSO), used to treat bladder problems and muscle pain, gives you garlic breath. Your body actually breaks down this drug into the chemical essence of garlic, then excretes it through your lungs and skin.
- Anticholinergic drugs, or drugs with anticholinergic effects, will dry out your mouth. They include antidepressants (for depression); antihistamines (for allergy); antipsychotics (for schizophrenia and other mental conditions); antiparkinsonians (for Parkinson's disease); and some drugs for intestinal problems, such as diarrhea.
- Diuretics, which remove excess fluid from your body, are often prescribed for high blood pressure and congestive heart failure. They also dry out your mouth.
- Antihypertensives, used to control high blood pressure, can give you dry mouth and bad breath.

When bad breath won't go away

Sometimes illnesses or diseases can cause bad breath. Read these symptoms carefully and see your doctor if you have any concerns.

Chronic kidney failure. If your breath constantly smells fishy or like ammonia and you have stomach pain, itchy skin, fatigue, paleness, muscle cramps and pain, tingling, and numbness or burning in your legs and feet, you might have chronic kidney failure.

Cirrhosis of the liver. This condition gives your breath a musty, rotten-egg odor. If you have mild jaundice, mental confusion, poor appetite and weight loss, fatigue and weakness, nausea or vomiting of blood, and excess fluid in your legs or abdomen, you could have cirrhosis of the liver. A history of hepatitis, liver damage, or alcohol consumption increases your risk.

Diabetic ketoacidosis. If you are diabetic, fruity-smelling breath could mean you have diabetic ketoacidosis, a dangerous condition in which your glucose level is severely out of balance. Other symptoms include stomach pain and tenderness, weakness, nausea and vomiting, and rapid heartbeat. This is a medical emergency, and you should get help immediately.

Lung condition or infection. A lung abscess, bronchitis, pneumonia, or emphysema can give you bad breath. Watch out for these warning signs — chronic cough with or without sputum, shortness of breath, fever and chills, and weight loss.

Periodontitis or tooth abscess. These serious dental problems can cause an unpleasant taste in your mouth and intense pain when chewing on the affected side. See your dentist as soon as possible to avoid tooth loss or an infection in your bloodstream.

Sinus infection. Constant bad breath, sinus drainage, headache, pain around your eyes and cheeks, and a general ill feeling could indicate a sinus infection.

Sjogren's syndrome. Bad breath caused by extreme dryness of your mouth and nasal passages can be an indication of Sjogren's syndrome. This autoimmune disease is common in people over the age of 50. This syndrome can also cause painful joints.

Bladder Infections

7 proven ways to beat bladder infections

Your doctor calls it cystitis. You may know it as a bladder infection. Whatever the name, once you've experienced the urgency, burning, tingling, and pain of a bladder infection, you don't ever want another one again.

Bladder infections, the most common type of urinary tract infections (UTIs), are the reason over 10 million women visit their doctors each year.

The bacteria that cause bladder infections, called E. coli, don't come from your urine because urine is sterile. That means it doesn't contain bacteria, viruses, or fungi. The bacteria get into your urethra, the tube urine travels through when it leaves your bladder, from your rectal area or skin. They travel up your urethra into your bladder, where they multiply, causing swelling, redness, and pain.

Most bladder infections can be prevented by following these tips.

Don't fight the urge. Go to the bathroom whenever you feel the need, and empty your bladder completely each time. You may be tempted to resist the urge to urinate if you're too busy to bother, or you think it's going to be painful. Just remember — the longer urine sits in your bladder, the more likely it is to stagnate and allow bacteria to grow.

Women should take special care to wipe from front to back. If you wipe from back to front, you may drag bacteria from your anus toward your urethra, giving germs a chance to set off an infection.

Urinate before and after sex. Emptying your bladder before and after sexual intercourse washes bacteria out of your urethra. It's also a good idea to wash your genital area before sex. This may help prevent spreading bacteria from one person to the other. If you use a diaphragm or if your partner uses a condom with spermicidal foam, research shows you are more likely to get urinary tract infections. Consider other forms of birth control.

Take a shower instead of a bath. Baths may be relaxing, but sitting in a tub of water may give bacteria an opportunity to enter your urethra. Take showers instead whenever possible. If your skin is sensitive, keep powders, soaps, creams, bath goods, or other hygiene products away from your genital area. Scented douches and feminine hygiene sprays may smell pretty, but they can also irritate your urethra.

Avoid foods that cause irritation. Certain foods and beverages may irritate your bladder. Common offenders include coffee, tea, alcohol, carbonated beverages, and spicy foods.

Drink cranberry juice. Although drinking lots of water is still sound advice for keeping your urinary tract healthy, cranberry juice is finally getting support from medical experts.

A study of two groups of women found that those who drank about 10 ounces of cranberry juice a day had fewer bladder infections than those who didn't. Researchers believe cranberry juice keeps bacteria from sticking to the walls of your urinary tract. Instead of hanging around, causing an infection, they are swept out of your body.

Stop smoking. In case you need another reason to ditch your cigarettes, smoking increases your risk for bladder infections.

Ask your doctor about new treatments. If you are postmenopausal, talk with your doctor about using a vaginal estrogen cream. It may help reduce the risk of urinary tract infections.

And be on the lookout for a vaccine against this common infection. Although still experimental, researchers hope it will prevent E. coli bacteria from attaching to the sides of your urinary tract and causing an infection.

If you end up with a bladder infection despite your best efforts, take care of it right away. That means seeing your doctor for a dose of antibiotics. Putting off treatment could allow the bacteria to travel to your kidneys or into your bloodstream, causing a more serious infection.

Frequent, painful urination, as well as fever, lower back pain, chills, nausea, and confusion, are symptoms of a kidney infection. An untreated kidney infection can cause permanent kidney damage.

Surprising cause of bladder infections

Some couples who figured Viagra would provide them with a second honeymoon are getting more than they bargained for. Cases of "honeymoon cystitis" — a painful condition experienced by some women after prolonged sexual activity — are now being reported by partners of Viagra users. This uncomfortable condition can cause:

► Painful, burning urination

► Frequent urination, or the feeling of having to urinate

► Excessive night urination

► Tenderness of pubic bone, sore pubic area

► Lower back pain

You should see your doctor as soon as these symptoms appear, although some of the discomfort can be relieved by drinking extra fluids and urinating before and after sex. If this doesn't help, your doctor can prescribe antibiotics to relieve the problem.

In the meantime, doctors stress the importance of avoiding sex, and Viagra, until the symptoms are gone.

Breast Cancer

Strengthen your defenses against breast cancer

Finding a lump in your breast can be frightening — with good reason. Each year about 43,000 women die from breast cancer. Early detection increases your chances of survival, which is why mammograms and monthly self-examinations are so important. But the best solution is preventing breast cancer in the first place.

In an attempt to find a way to prevent breast cancer, researchers conducted the Breast Cancer Prevention Trial. This huge study concluded that tamoxifen, a drug used to treat breast cancer, could also help prevent it in women at high risk.

Unfortunately, tamoxifen may also increase your risk of cataracts, double your risk of uterine cancer, and triple your risk of life-threatening blood clots. Whether or not you should take it depends on how likely you are to get breast cancer.

The decision to use tamoxifen as a breast cancer preventive is so complicated the National Cancer Institute developed a software program designed to help you and your doctor compute your risks. If you are in a high-risk category for breast cancer, ask your doctor about tamoxifen and the assessment program provided by the NCI.

In the meantime, there are several things you can do to reduce your risk of breast cancer:

Watch your weight. Adult weight gain, particularly after menopause, can increase your risk of breast cancer. After menopause, your body gets estrogen from body fat. The more weight you gain, the more estrogen circulating in your body, which contributes to your breast cancer risk. In one large study, women who had never been on hormone replacement therapy and who gained at least 45 pounds were about twice as likely to get breast cancer after menopause than women who had gained only a few pounds.

Pick your fats wisely. A low-fat diet can help prevent weight gain, which increases your risk of breast cancer. However, the types of fat you choose to eat can also play a role in whether you develop the disease. A recent study found that monounsaturated fats, found in olive and canola oils, reduced the risk of breast cancer by 45 percent, while polyunsaturated fats, found in corn, safflower, and sunflower oils, increased the risk by 69 percent. Saturated fats, found in meat and dairy products, had no effect on breast cancer risk in this study.

Munch on fresh fruits and veggies. Eating a diet rich in fruits and vegetables may reduce your risk of breast cancer and other cancers. One study found that eating carrots and spinach more than twice a week were particularly associated with a lower risk of breast cancer. Another study found that supplements of vitamins C, E, and folic acid had no effect on risk, while eating vegetables had a strong protective effect. This means vitamin supplements may be a poor substitute for fresh fruits and vegetables. According to the researchers, several different components in fruits and vegetables may work together to help provide protection.

Drink your milk. Women need plenty of calcium to help keep their bones strong, but one study suggests that drinking milk may do more than provide you with calcium. It could help you avoid breast cancer. The study found that there was a significant decrease in breast cancer risk between women who drank the most milk and women who drank the least. In this study, other dairy foods didn't have the same protective effect.

Pass on the alcohol. Drinking even small amounts of alcohol every day may contribute to breast cancer risk. In a recent study, women who drank even one drink a day were more likely to develop invasive breast cancer. Those who drank two to five alcoholic drinks a day were 41 percent more likely to get breast cancer than those who didn't drink alcohol at all.

Try some flaxseed. The American Institute for Cancer Research is funding a study on the effects of flaxseed on breast cancer risk. While the results of the research aren't in yet, this nutty little seed shows a lot of promise in helping to prevent the disease. Flaxseed is high in healthful omega-3 fatty acids, vitamin D, and fiber. Adding a little to your diet would be a healthy and tasty change.

Breast cancer risk factors

- **Age.** Most breast cancers occur in women over age 50.
- **Family history.** If you have a mother, daughter, or sister who has had breast cancer, your chances of getting it increase.
- **Personal history.** If you've had breast cancer in one breast, you're more likely to get it again.
- **Age at first menstrual period.** If you began menstruating before age 12, your risk increases.
- **Late childbirth.** Having your first child after age 30, or not having children at all, increases your risk.
- **Late menopause.** If you go through menopause after age 55, your risk increases.

Eat a cherry burger to lower breast cancer risk

If you're concerned about breast cancer, pass up the steak at dinner and eat some broccoli. Fruits and veggies can help reduce your risk of breast cancer, and they may do double duty if they also help you eat less red meat. According to a recent study, women who ate the most red meat had a 78 percent higher risk of breast cancer than those who ate the least.

How you like your meat cooked can also make a difference. Women who liked their meat well-done — charred or heavily browned — had a four times greater risk of developing breast cancer than women who preferred their meat rare or medium. But don't eat meat that's undercooked, or you could end up with food poisoning.

Researchers say chemicals called heterocyclic aromatic amines (HAAs) are formed on the surface of meat during high-temperature cooking. In a recent study, these chemicals were shown to cause cancer.

But a tiny fruit may help you have your meat and eat it, too. When researchers added cherries to hamburger meat, it resulted in significantly fewer HAAs. And the cherry burgers were moist and juicy, even though the fat content of the burgers was lower than regular burgers. Several states already offer cherry burgers on their school menus.

The next time you simply must have a burger — make it a cherry burger.

Mammograms and heart disease

You know mammograms can detect breast cancer while it's still treatable, and yet you put off getting one. Well, now you have another reason to make that appointment and get a mammogram — they may also detect heart disease.

A recent study found that women with breast arterial calcification (BAC) were 35 percent more likely to die of heart disease than women without BAC. Fortunately, BAC, which is an accumulation of calcium in the arteries of your breast, shows up on a mammogram.

At your next appointment, ask your doctor to request that your mammogram be checked for BAC as well as breast tumors.

Burns

Banish burns from your kitchen

The next time you're racing around your kitchen trying to get dinner ready, remember this. Cooking fires are the leading cause of fires in the home. And burns are the second leading cause of accidental death.

If you are an older person, especially one with poor vision or arthritis, you need to take extra precautions. You can prevent most burns by thinking ahead and following these tips.

- ▶ Don't wear loose clothing when using the stove. Bathrobes with long, floppy sleeves are especially dangerous.

- ▶ Wear clothing you can remove quickly if it catches fire. Dresses and tops that open down the front and have Velcro fasteners rather than buttons are easier to get out of safely.

- ▶ If your clothing catches fire, stop, sit down, and calmly pat out the fire. Frantic movements can fan the flames and make your injuries worse.

- ▶ Cook on an electric rather than a gas stove to avoid the danger of flames. Use plug-in appliances, like tea kettles and small ovens, instead of the stove when possible.

- ▶ Be careful of food cooked in a microwave oven. It can be cool on the surface but scalding hot in the middle. Containers, too, can feel comfortable to the touch, while the food inside may be burning hot.

- ▶ To prevent scalding from hot water, have a plumber or electrician lower the temperature setting on your water heater. Most are set at 140 degrees. Water that hot can cause a third degree burn — the worst kind — in only five seconds. At 120 degrees, it takes three minutes of contact to do the same.

Adults over age 60 get burned more often than younger adults, and their burns tend to be larger as well. With care, you can avoid most of them. But if you do burn yourself, get help immediately. If you're alone, call 911.

Sure-fire burn remedies

The pan slips as you are taking your favorite chocolate chip cookies out of the oven. Without thinking, you grab it with your bare hand. Ouch!

Before you do anything else, run cold water over the burn. Cold water helps relieve the pain. It's also the best way to stop the burning, which prevents damage to the skin and deeper layers of tissue.

Continue holding the burn under the running water — or press a cold, wet cloth to the area — until the pain goes away. It may take from 10 to 45 minutes.

If you get a burn and water isn't available, use any cold liquid that's clean enough to drink.

Once you've cooled your injury, you need to decide if you should see a doctor. Here are some guidelines to help you. They come from Dr. Scott Dinehart, dermatologist and associate professor in the Department of Dermatology at the University of Arkansas.

- ▶ **Pay attention to how you feel.** Serious burns can affect you all over, not just where you were injured. "If you get a burn," says Dinehart, "and as a result are feeling sick — running a fever or just feeling bad in general — that would be a good sign to see a physician."

- ▶ **Beware of blisters.** If you get a single blister, you probably don't need to worry. But if you get a lot of water-filled bubbles at the site of the burn, Dinehart suggests a visit to your doctor.

- ▶ **Size up the injury.** A burn the size of your palm or bigger may be serious. Call your doctor.

- ▶ **Watch out for danger signals.** "If you see signs of infection, like extreme warmth around the area, fever, or pus, you want to check with your physician," says Dinehart.

If you require medical care, your doctor may prescribe medication. For less serious burns, Dinehart says NSAIDs (nonsteroidal anti-inflammatory drugs), like aspirin or ibuprofen, can help relieve symptoms and decrease inflammation.

To care for your burn, wash it gently with a mild soap and warm water and coat it with an antibiotic cream. Never put butter or any other nonsterile grease on your burn. Cover the burned area lightly with gauze. Wash the burn and change the dressing once or twice a day.

Don't pop a blister. It's nature's way of protecting the burned tissue. If one does break, cover the area with a thin layer of antibiotic ointment.

The pros and cons of herbal relief

Even though many herbal preparations are used on burns, Dr. Scott Dinehart says most haven't been tested, at least not on humans. While some have stood the test of time as well as scientific study, others, he warns, can be dangerous.

▶ **Bromelain.** Dinehart says this herbal remedy may be useful for burns because it reduces swelling. "And," he says, "it's relatively inexpensive." You can buy it over-the-counter at drugstores and supermarkets. Bromelain comes from the pineapple. If you're wondering if eating the fruit would help your burn, Dinehart doesn't think so. "Bromelain actually comes from the stem of the pineapple," he says. "It doesn't come from the fruit. So there's no reason to think that would help." There are no known side effects, but if you are allergic to pineapple, you might want to pass up the bromelain.

▶ **Aloe.** Inside the thick, fleshy leaves of the aloe plant, you'll find a soothing gel. You might want to keep an aloe plant in your kitchen window for minor burns and other small injuries. Just break off a piece and squeeze the cooling jelly-like sap onto your burned skin. Not only can it relieve pain, prevent blistering, and reduce swelling, it may also prevent scarring.

▶ **Comfrey.** This controversial herb, also called knitbone, is sometimes used as a poultice to heal burns, as well as sprains, swellings, and bruises. Dinehart says taking it internally can cause cancer or liver damage. Until its safety and effectiveness have been established, he doesn't advise using comfrey in any form. "Topically, it hasn't been a miracle," he says. "And because it's such a big problem internally, we don't recommend people have it around at all."

Dinehart would like to see more testing of herbal remedies. He encourages people to lobby the Food and Drug Administration (FDA) for more regulation of herbal products.

How severe is your burn?

First-degree burns. These are the least serious, involving only the outer layer of skin. The affected area is usually red but turns white when you touch it. There may be mild swelling, tenderness, and pain. These burns generally leave no scars. Sunburn is the most common first-degree burn.

Second-degree burns. These extend through the outer layer and into the inner layer of skin. They may appear white, or white with some redness, and look wet or waxy. You might experience blisters, swelling, and a lot of pain.

These burns are often caused by flames, oil, or grease and usually leave a scar. You may find it difficult to tell the difference between second-degree and third-degree burns.

Third-degree burns. These are the most serious kind because they penetrate all skin layers. They may even damage underlying fat and muscle tissue. Your skin may look gray-white or charred, perhaps leathery. If you press on the burn, it won't look whiter as it does with first-degree burns.

With third-degree burns, the nerve endings are destroyed, so you may feel pressure instead of pain. If you have a third-degree burn, get medical attention right away.

Carpal Tunnel Syndrome

Protect your wrists from strain and pain

Variety is the spice of life. Never is that saying more true than for someone suffering from carpal tunnel syndrome. If your work or hobby involves repeating a certain motion with your hands, tendons in your wrist can swell, pinching a nerve and causing pain. Changing the way you do things will not only spice up your life, it might prevent wrist pain.

There are many names for it — tendonitis, repetitive motion injury, cumulative trauma disorder. Whether you type, sew, drive a bus, cut hair, operate power tools, or play a musical instrument, you are at risk.

You might have carpal tunnel syndrome if your fingers, hands, or wrists become weak; you have numbness, tingling, or burning in your hands or fingers; or you have pain that travels up your arm, especially at night.

Some people resort to surgery to ease the pressure on the nerve, but surgery has side effects and very often the symptoms reappear. Your best plan is to prevent carpal tunnel syndrome in the first place.

Try a wrist workout. Experts from the American Academy of Orthopaedic Surgeons say carpal tunnel syndrome can be prevented by regularly stretching and exercising your wrists. They advise you to get in the habit of doing exercises like these several times a day.

▶ Take a break every hour and vigorously shake your hands for about 15 seconds. This relieves cramped muscles and gets your blood flowing.

▶ Hold your arms straight out in front of you, palms down. Bend your wrists up until your palms are facing front and you feel a nice easy stretch in your forearms. Repeat this several times.

▶ Make your hand into a tight fist. Bend your wrist down to stretch your forearm. Straighten your wrist and open up your hand, fanning your fingers out as far apart as possible. Hold and repeat several times.

▶ Sit with your forearm resting on the arm of your chair. With your opposite hand, grab your fingers and pull so your wrist is gently stretched back. Hold this position for about 15 seconds. Then let your wrist relax so your fingers are pointing toward the ground. Gently push on the back of your hand so your wrist and forearm are stretched down. Hold for 15 seconds. Repeat several times with each hand.

Watch how you sit. The majority of people suffering from carpal tunnel syndrome spend many hours at a computer. Although there are hundreds of products designed for computer users to ease wrist strain, such as ergonomic keyboards, mice, and wrist supports, some experts think this near-epidemic of wrist injury is due to how you sit, not the position of your hands.

No matter what you are doing, when you sit, your body posture naturally follows how your head and upper arms are positioned. Keeping them in line with your spine and hips forces your back, shoulders, abdomen, forearms, and hands to stay in a stress-free position.

When you're sitting, whether it's in front of a computer or a sewing machine, don't let your head or upper arms reach forward. Keep your chest directly over your pelvis, with your diaphragm and stomach muscles tightened and lifted.

When you are using a keyboard, your weight should not be on your wrists. This only increases the pressure on the nerves in your wrist. That's why wrist supports may not relieve carpal tunnel syndrome. If your body is positioned properly, you won't need to support your wrists at all. They will simply glide over the keys with an easy, relaxed arm motion.

Be kind to your wrists. Remember, you don't have to sit in front of a computer to suffer from carpal tunnel syndrome. It can come from any activity that involves doing the same thing over and over again with your hands. Even something as relaxing as gardening or woodworking can cause this physical stress. To avoid turning a favorite pastime into a painful chore, follow these wrist-saving tips:

► Change tasks every 30 minutes.

► Take a break between tasks. Run through a few of the hand exercises mentioned previously.

► Don't lean your weight on your hands. Work in a position where your body weight is supported by stronger joints.

► Buy tools that have padded handles or are ergonomically designed.

► Put shock absorbers on power tools.

► Try to keep your grip on objects as loose and relaxed as possible.

► Change positions frequently.

► Use electrical devices that will save your hands, like power staplers, tillers, etc.

► Use as little force as possible to get the job done. Typing with a light touch can correct carpal tunnel syndrome.

Soothe wrist pain with yoga

If your doctor prescribes a wrist splint for your carpal tunnel, tell him to hold everything. A study at the University of Pennsylvania School of Medicine showed that practicing simple yoga postures twice a week can improve grip strength and flexibility and reduce numbness and pain better than wearing a wrist splint.

Try these nine yoga postures that concentrate on stretching your joints and increasing blood flow.

Dandasana. Sit on the floor against a wall (or on a chair) with your body straight and tall. Press the palms of your hands down onto the floor beside your hips. Press your shoulder blades against the wall and feel the top of your head lifting toward the ceiling. Hold for 30 seconds. Breathe comfortably through your nose.

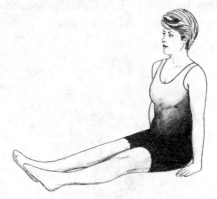

Namaste. Bend your elbows and lift them out and away from the sides of your body. Press your palms and fingers together with your fingers spread as widely as possible. Hold this pressure for 30 seconds. Then press each "set" of fingers individually. Hold each press for 30 seconds. Breathe through your nose.

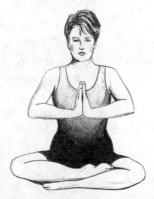

Garudasana. Stand straight and well-balanced. Bend your elbows and cross your arms in front of your chest so your left elbow rests on the inside bend of your right arm. Circle your right hand in toward your chest, counterclockwise, so your right fingers rest against your left palm. Your elbows should be shoulder level. Stretch your hands and fingers toward the ceiling. Hold for 30 seconds. Release and repeat by reversing the position of your arms.

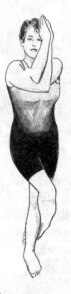

Bharadvajasana. Sit sideways on a chair so your right hip and thigh are against the back of the chair. Keep breathing and lengthen your spine with your shoulders down and back. Twist your upper body to the right so you can place your hands on the back of the chair. Use your hands to gently increase the pressure of the twist — push against the chair with your right hand and pull with your left. Look over your right shoulder. Hold for 30 seconds, relax, then repeat on the left side.

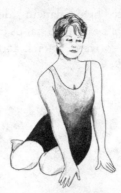

Tadasana. Stand barefoot with your feet together and your weight evenly balanced. Tighten your thigh muscles so your kneecaps lift. Lengthen your spine, drop your shoulders, and raise your chest. Keeping your arms at your side, rotate your upper arms outward so your palms are facing as far back as possible. Hold for 30 seconds, breathing evenly through your nose.

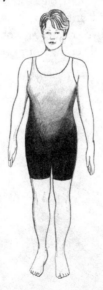

Half Uttanasana. Stand with your feet about shoulder-width apart. Either place your hands on your hips or stretch them over your head. Keeping your spine straight, bend at the waist as far as you comfortably can. If you need help balancing, do this in front of a wall or the back of a chair so your extended hands end up against the wall or chair back as you bend forward. Stretch and hold for 30 seconds.

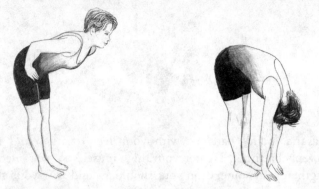

Virabhadrasana (arms only). Stand with your feet about shoulder-width apart. Lift your arms out from your sides until they are shoulder high then rotate them back so your palms are facing up. Raise them over your head until your palms are touching and your elbows are slightly behind your ears. Stretch your arms and fingers to the ceiling. Lift your chest, keeping your shoulders down and relaxed. Hold for 30 seconds.

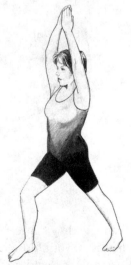

Urdhva Mukha Svanasana. Lie face down on the floor. Place your hands under your shoulders with your fingers spread wide. Straighten your elbows so just your chest and upper body are lifted off the floor. Push the heels of your hands into the floor. Keep your head level and your shoulders down and back. Breathe evenly. Hold this stretch for 30 seconds.

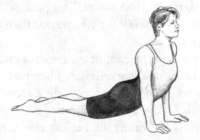

Savasana. Lie flat on your back so your body is straight. Rest your arms slightly away from your body with the palms up. Your heels should be about hip-distance apart. Relax your feet so your toes fall out to the sides. Close your eyes and relax all your muscles. Breathe deeply. Remain in this position for about 10 minutes.

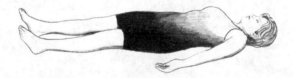

Silence carpal tunnel pain with ultrasound

Treating carpal tunnel syndrome can be frustrating. Conventional remedies, like steroid injections and wearing a splint at night, don't always work. Surgery is an option, but it doesn't work for everyone. Now carpal tunnel sufferers have another choice — ultrasound treatments.

Ultrasound is the use of high-frequency sound waves, those beyond the range of normal hearing, to treat injuries to ligaments, muscles, and tendons. It can reduce inflammation and speed up healing by improving blood flow through your tissues. You may feel warmth or tingling during an ultrasound treatment but rarely any pain.

Researchers at the University of Vienna tested ultrasound treatments on 34 patients with carpal tunnel syndrome. The study lasted seven weeks with a six-month follow-up. The patients received 15-minute treatments five days a week for two weeks, then twice a week for another five weeks.

At the end of this time, 68 percent of the patients said their symptoms were improved or completely relieved. They had less pain and numbness, greater hand strength, and no side effects. Even better news, at the six-month follow-up, the number of satisfied patients had risen to 74 percent. This means the healing effects of ultrasound last beyond the original treatments.

If you're interested in this latest therapy, talk with your doctor to see if it's right for you.

Cataracts

7 ways to steer clear of cataracts

Good nutrition and a healthy lifestyle will not only lower your risk of heart disease and cancer, they may protect your eyes from cataracts — the leading cause of blindness.

A cataract is a cloudy area in the lens. When it's small, it has little effect on vision. As the cataract grows, you may notice that your vision is blurred, like looking through a cloudy piece of glass. Light from the sun or a lamp may seem too bright, causing a glare. When you drive at night, you may notice that the oncoming headlights cause more glare than before. Colors may appear faded.

Most cataracts develop naturally as you age. Half of all Americans have cataracts by age 50, and by age 75 that number increases to 70 percent. Cataract surgery usually improves vision, but sometimes stronger reading glasses or better light when doing close work is all you need.

Even so, wouldn't you rather stay in that smaller group — the 30 percent that never get cataracts? Making these healthy choices can help keep cloudy lenses from spoiling your view.

Fight back with antioxidants. Antioxidants help prevent cataracts by fighting free radicals, which can damage your eyes. Try getting more of these three powerful antioxidants every day to prevent vision loss.

▶ **Beta carotene.** Found in dark green and bright orange foods like carrots, sweet potatoes, apricots, broccoli, and spinach, beta carotene converts to vitamin A in your body. Since too much vitamin A can be dangerous, it's best to get this nutrient from foods rather than supplements. But if you have a hard time eating those deep-colored vegetables, taking a daily multiple vitamin will supply all you need. In fact, research shows that taking a multiple vitamin each day may lower your risk of developing cataracts.

▶ **Vitamin E.** A recent study found that nuclear cataracts, the most common kind, grow twice as fast in people who don't take vitamin E supplements when compared with people who do. Some researchers say you can safely take up to 400 international units (IU) of vitamin E daily in supplement form. To get more vitamin E in your diet, add a little wheat germ oil, sunflower seeds, or dried almonds. Instead of white flour and white rice, eat whole wheat, oats, and brown rice.

▶ **Vitamin C.** Researchers conducted a study of nurses between the ages of 56 and 71. They found that those who took a vitamin C supplement for 10 years or more were 77 percent less likely to have even mild clouding of the lenses than those who weren't taking supplements. It seems the amount of vitamin C in the supplement is less important than the number of years you take it. The advantage wasn't as great for those who took it for less than 10 years. To get more vitamin C from food, eat oranges, lemons, tangerines, strawberries, broccoli, brussels sprouts, and sweet red peppers.

Savor an exotic spice. Curcumin, a natural antioxidant found in the spice turmeric, may help prevent cataracts. Turmeric is an essential ingredient of curry powder, which is used in Indian cooking. Give this flavorful spice a try — your taste buds will thank you and so will your eyes.

Go easy on the salt. If you are salt-sensitive, too much salt in your diet can cause your blood pressure to rise and interfere with the blood vessels in your eyes. Most people should limit their salt intake to 2,400 milligrams (mg) a day. If you have high blood pressure, don't get more than 2,000 mg. Learn to cook without salt. Use spices to add a little zing to your meals. Make wise choices when eating out, and read labels for sodium content when you're at the grocery store.

Think low-fat. Protecting your eyes is another reason to eat less fat. To keep your daily fat calories to 30 percent or less, avoid fried foods, choose low-fat versions of your favorite high-fat foods, and use a nonstick cooking spray when preparing meals. If you eat more fruits, vegetables, and whole grains, you'll automatically eat less fat.

Throw away your cigarettes. Cigarette smoke can do more than cloud up a room. It can dim your eyesight as well. Smokers are two to three times more likely to get cataracts than nonsmokers.

Wear sunglasses with UV protection. Avoid spending too much time in bright sunlight. When you go outside, wear sunglasses and a wide brimmed hat and stay in the shade. This is especially important if you live near the equator or at a high elevation.

Ask your doctor about aspirin. Some studies have indicated that taking aspirin might help prevent cataracts. But more recent evidence shows long-term use of aspirin can actually increase your risk. Researchers found that people who took one or more aspirin tablets a week for a period of 10 years were twice as likely to have cataracts as those who didn't take aspirin very often. This seemed to be truest for people under age 65.

A word of caution — if you are taking aspirin for your heart or other health reasons, don't stop without your doctor's approval.

How to buy sunglasses

You probably think wearing sunglasses makes you look cool. But sunglasses are more than a fashion statement — they're essential for the health of your eyes.

Don't be confused by the many styles, colors, materials, prices, and advertising claims. Consider these basics before you buy:

Sunglasses should block ultraviolet light. Check the label to be sure the glasses cut off 99 to 100 percent of all ultraviolet light (both UV-A and UV-B). If the label says "UV absorption up to 400 nm," that means the same thing.

Don't worry about protection from infrared light. Research hasn't shown any connection between eye problems and the relatively low levels found in sunlight.

Large, wrap-around styles stop more rays. Ordinary frames allow light to shine around the sides, over the tops, and into your eyes. These provide protection from all angles.

Quality can vary. Nonprescription sunglasses that are ground and polished by the manufacturer are generally of better quality. On the other hand, those that aren't won't hurt your eyes.

To judge the quality of sunglasses, it helps to look at something with a rectangular pattern — perhaps floor tile. Holding the glasses several inches from your face, cover one eye, and move the glasses from side to side and up and down. The lines should stay straight. If they look wavy, especially in the center, look for another pair.

Expensive doesn't mean better. It isn't necessary to pay big bucks for good sunglasses. That $100 pair may have more style, but the $10 pair could be just as good, or better, for your eyes. Remember — UV protection is what matters most, not the price.

Cervical Cancer

Maximize your defenses against cervical cancer

Cervical cancer is a sneaky, slow-growing cancer with almost no symptoms. It's possible to never know you have it until it's too late. Scary stuff. But there's something you can do to lower your risk of getting this cancer — eat more fruits and vegetables.

A diet lacking in vitamins and minerals causes your immune system to become too weak to resist illness and disease. Experts have proven that fruits and vegetables are the most important food group for fighting many kinds of cancer. And one nutrient may be more important than others in the war on cervical cancer. It's folic acid, one of the B vitamins.

When researchers at the University of Illinois compared a group of women with cervical cancer to a group without cervical cancer, they found the noncancerous group had a higher level of folic acid in their diets. Their conclusion — more folic acid may mean less cervical cancer.

The recommended dietary allowance (RDA) for folic acid is 400 micrograms (mcg) a day. You can meet your day's quota with just one cup of cooked lentils and a fresh spinach salad.

If you use supplements, don't go overboard. Experts say you shouldn't get more than 1 milligram (mg) of folic acid a day. Your best food sources are legumes; enriched whole grain products, like cereals, pasta, bread, and rice; citrus fruits; berries; and dark green leafy vegetables.

Now that you're eating healthy, your second line of defense is early detection. If caught early enough, cervical cancer is almost 100 percent curable. The best way to detect it is with a screening test called the Pap smear. Health professionals recommend women have a pelvic exam and Pap smear every one to three years. The test involves taking a sample of cells from around your cervix and sending it to a lab for analysis. This simple procedure has caused the number of deaths from cervical cancer to drop 74 percent in the last 40 years.

Remember these other high risk factors — smoking, numerous sexual partners, oral contraceptives, and having many children. If you feel you are at risk, don't wait. See your doctor for a Pap smear, and pick up some spinach on the way.

Cholesterol

Clobber cholesterol with these natural strategies

Your body needs cholesterol. It's a building block of the outer membrane of cells; it's a principal ingredient of bile, a fluid that helps with digestion; it's present in the fatty sheath that insulates nerves; and it helps with the production of hormones.

Most of the cholesterol in your body is produced in the liver, but 20 to 30 percent comes from the food you eat. Too much cholesterol can clog your arteries and lead to heart disease and stroke.

If your cholesterol levels are high, talk with your doctor about cholesterol therapy, and try these natural cholesterol-lowering strategies.

Flatten your "spare tire." If you are overweight, drop those extra pounds. Losing weight, especially around your middle, lowers your triglycerides and bad LDL cholesterol and raises your good HDL cholesterol. This reduces your risk of heart disease. Exercise can do the same thing. If you exercise and lose weight, you'll increase your HDL even more.

Pick your fats wisely. There are three kinds of fats — saturated, polyunsaturated, and monounsaturated.

Saturated fats raise your cholesterol level. They are found in meat, egg yolks, cream, milk, butter, and cheese, as well as a few vegetable fats like coconut oil, palm oil, and hydrogenated vegetable shortenings.

Polyunsaturated fats lower LDL cholesterol, which is good, but they also lower HDL cholesterol, which is bad. A little of this kind of fat in your diet is OK — just don't overdo it. Safflower oil, sunflower oil, and soybean oil are high in polyunsaturates.

Monounsaturated fats lower LDL cholesterol and can raise HDL cholesterol. Olive oil and canola oil are high in monounsaturated fats. Study after study has proven that olive oil lowers bad LDL cholesterol and raises good HDL cholesterol. In fact, adding olive oil to a low-fat diet produces better results than just cutting out fat.

Eat less fat. Your body needs some fat. It's one of your best sources of energy, it's necessary for growth, and it carries the fat-soluble vitamins A, D, E, and K throughout your body. And did you know a little fat actually helps to curb your appetite? That's why a very low-fat diet may make you feel hungry all the time.

The U.S. Department of Health and Human Services recommends a total dietary fat intake of no more than 30 percent of your total calories. That means if you are on a 2,000 calorie-a-day diet, you should not eat more than 600 fat calories a day. And keep your saturated fat intake as low as possible. The American Heart Association says saturated fat should be no more than 7 percent of your total daily calories. If you don't like to keep track of numbers, simply cut out high-fat foods or eat the low-fat versions.

Feast on fiber. Fiber helps lower bad LDL cholesterol and may even raise good HDL cholesterol. Fiber also fills you up, leaving less room for meat and dairy products high in cholesterol and fats. Bran, oats, barley, wild rice, hominy, and flaxseed are good sources of fiber. Legumes, like split peas, black-eyed peas, lentils, kidney beans, and soybeans are another inexpensive way to add fiber to your meals. And don't forget fruits and vegetables. They make great snacks and are loaded with fiber.

Give butter the heave-ho. Butter is high in cholesterol and saturated fat. Margarine, on the other hand, is usually made from unsaturated liquid vegetable oil, and it doesn't have cholesterol. But margarine isn't perfect. When vegetable oils are hardened during hydrogenation, trans fatty acids are formed. Research shows that trans fatty acids are as bad for your cholesterol as saturated fats.

To help you make a choice, consider the latest American Heart Association recommendations:

▶ Choose a margarine with no more than 2 grams of saturated fat per tablespoon.

▶ Look for a margarine with liquid vegetable oil listed as the first ingredient.

▶ Buy soft margarines instead of stick.

And how about two new margarine substitutes that help lower cholesterol? One is made from sitostanol ester, a by-product of the wood processing industry. Studies show this margarine resulted in a 20 percent drop in LDL cholesterol by blocking absorption of some cholesterol into the bloodstream. It is marketed by Johnson & Johnson under the brand name Benecol.

Another heart-healthy spread is made from plant sterols extracted from soybeans. This one, called Take Control, is a Lipton foods product.

Don't be afraid of eggs. Egg yolks have taken a beating lately because they contain cholesterol. The American Heart Association recommends that most people limit their intake of cholesterol to 300 milligrams (mg) per day, and the average large egg contains about 213 to 220 mg of cholesterol.

This doesn't have to mean the end of French toast and omelets. Go ahead and indulge in that three-egg omelet for Sunday brunch as long as you cut back on meat and whole dairy products the rest of the week. In fact, the American Heart Association says about four egg yolks a week is all right for people with normal cholesterol. The tricky part is counting the hidden eggs in your food. One serving of a baked good counts as one-half an egg yolk.

Munch on some garlic. This small, unassuming herb, which has been used in cooking and healing for thousands of years, can put the spring back into your arteries.

There are dozens of studies showing that garlic prevents the build-up of fat and cholesterol in your arteries, reduces triglycerides, and increases HDL cholesterol. In one of those studies, eating a fresh clove of garlic every day for 16 weeks reduced cholesterol by an amazing 20 percent.

If cholesterol is a concern for you, plan a few meals around garlic and fatty fish, like salmon. This combination seems to lower cholesterol better than either one alone.

Get some vitamin C. Studies find that vitamin C raises HDL cholesterol, and it helps prevent LDL cholesterol from becoming oxidized and turning into artery-clogging plaques.

The recommended dietary allowance (RDA) for vitamin C is 75 milligrams (mg) daily for women and 90 mg daily for men. Just a glass of orange juice will do the trick. Some other good sources of vitamin C are sweet red peppers, green peppers, kiwifruit, strawberries, cantaloupe, brussels sprouts, tomato juice, grapefruit, collard greens, broccoli, and cabbage.

The Asian diet — humble eating for a healthy heart

It took the largest study of its kind, but the results are undeniable. If you want to live longer and healthier, eat like an Asian peasant.

Researchers have known for some time that people living in countries like China, Japan, Thailand, India, Korea, and Indonesia have a lower risk of cancer, obesity, and heart disease. They just never had the hard evidence to tell them why. Now they do.

In a Chinese diet study, called the China-Cornell-Oxford Diet and Health Project, researchers have been collecting information on the eating habits of over 10,000 Chinese since 1983. They've found that the lower class "peasant" Asians eat a humble, traditional diet — full of high-fiber grains and vegetables, with few animal products. This, they say, is the reason for their good health. Cholesterol levels are low — so low in fact that their average high cholesterol is still about equal to the lowest range in the United States. And only an average of 15 percent of deaths in Asia are due to heart disease, compared with more than 40 percent in the United States.

The super heart-saving Asian diet has won the approval of many nutrition experts because it emphasizes plant-based, rather than animal-based, foods. Following this type of eating pattern may be your path to sound health and a long life.

Here are the basic groups that make up the Asian food pyramid. There are many ways to include these foods in your everyday eating without having to give up your own traditions. On the other hand, if you're tired of the same old meat and potatoes routine, why not buy a Chinese cookbook and learn the art of stir-frying.

Grains. Most of your diet should consist of unrefined rice, wheat, millet, corn, barley, and other grains. Other dishes are generally eaten alongside, but only in small amounts, to add variety and zest. Look for unpolished rice, basmati, jasmine, or brown rice. They are full of flavor, fragrance, and fiber.

Vegetables. Whether from the land or the sea, vegetables play a big part in the everyday Asian diet. Some that you may find in traditional Asian recipes are bok choy, Chinese mustard greens, amaranth, water spinach, water chestnuts, bamboo shoots, lotus root, and bitter melon. However, vegetables like broccoli, spinach, celery, carrots, and peppers are easily adapted to traditional Asian recipes.

Legumes. Peas and beans are a huge source of fiber and protein. They should be part of at least one meal a day. Besides soybeans, other legumes you can try for an authentic Asian taste are mung beans, chickpeas, and lentils.

Nuts and seeds. Almonds, cashews, walnuts, pine nuts, and chestnuts are all popular ingredients in Asian cooking. Many are crushed and mixed with water to form nut milk, which is then used in sauces, desserts, and dressings. Try to get about a handful of nuts or seeds every day.

Fats and oils. Small amounts of peanut, golden sesame, soy, and corn oils may be eaten daily.

Seafood. Although it's often more expensive than chicken or red meat, fish is worth the extra pennies. It's full of omega-3 fatty acids and protein, but low in cholesterol.

Meat. To help keep your arteries healthy, some experts recommend eating red meat only once a month and cutting back on poultry and eggs — no more than an average serving each week.

Herbs. No eating plan would be complete without the herbs and spices unique to that culture. Many not only add flavor and spice to the food, but some, like garlic, turmeric, and fenugreek, provide powerful heart protection, too.

Sweets. If you want to follow the Asian diet, you must cut back on sugar and sweets. In Asia, fresh fruits, not sweets, are served for dessert.

Ketchup gives bad cholesterol the boot

A hot dog might not do your heart any favors, but what you put on top just might. Some studies have shown that lycopene, which is found naturally in tomatoes, can lower your risk of heart disease and certain types of cancer. But according to a recent study, the best source of lycopene is not tomatoes, it's ketchup.

Research endorsed by the Cancer Research Foundation of America reveals that cooked tomatoes, like those used to make ketchup, provide as much as five times more lycopene than fresh tomatoes.

This natural antioxidant protects your heart by preventing the oxidation of bad LDL cholesterol in your arteries. Lycopene doesn't lessen the amount of cholesterol in your blood. It just keeps the cholesterol from doing any damage.

In one study at the University of Toronto, people were given one-to-two servings per day of tomato-based products, such as tomato juice, spaghetti sauce, and concentrated lycopene. After just one week, lycopene levels were doubled in the participants and their levels of oxidized LDL cholesterol went down significantly.

So how much ketchup do you need to reap these great benefits? Getting about 40 milligrams (mg) of lycopene a day is enough to give you a leg up in the fight against heart disease. Unfortunately, you'd have to drown your hot dog in about a cup of ketchup to get this much. But there are other good ways to get lycopene. Almost anything tomato-based is a rich source. Just two cups of tomato juice or 3/4 cup of spaghetti sauce will do the trick. You can also get lycopene from guava, watermelon, rosehip, and pink grapefruit.

Perilla packs a healthy punch

Omega-3 fatty acids help lower LDL cholesterol and raise HDL cholesterol. Fish that live in cold, deep waters, like salmon, tuna, and sardines, are rich sources of omega-3. Omega-3 is also found in flaxseed, walnuts, and oat germ but in lesser amounts.

Now a vegetable oil used for centuries in the East is gaining popularity in the West. It's called perilla oil, and it's extremely high in omega-3 fatty acids. Even better, it doesn't give you the stomach and intestinal distress that sometimes goes with other oils high in omega-3.

Perilla oil comes from the beefsteak plant (Perilla frutescens). It looks like coleus and is a cousin of mint. In the early 20th century, it was popular as an ornamental plant. Its seed oil has been used in varnish, paint, linoleum, lacquer, and ink, but don't worry — it has also been used for cooking in Korean kitchens for generations. Fresh perilla leaves, called "shiso," are used as garnish in Japanese dishes and enjoyed for their delicate flavor and fragrance. The plant has also been used in the Orient for years as a medicinal herb.

Researchers are looking into the specific benefits of perilla oil for treating cancer, heart disease, allergies, obesity, and intestinal diseases, as well as enhancing brain function.

Your best bet for finding perilla oil today is in an Oriental grocery store, a natural foods store, or on the Internet.

The jury is still out on perilla as a drug. But for now, perilla oil seems to be another good choice for adding omega-3 to your diet.

Chronic Pain

Surgery-free solution for chronic pain

Are you in constant pain? Have you given up hope of ever swinging a tennis racket, walking through the park, or simply getting a good night's sleep? If so, prolotherapy, a revolutionary treatment, may help relieve or even cure your chronic pain while making your body stronger and more stable — all without drugs or surgery.

Since prolotherapy was first developed in the 1950s, thousands of people have been successfully treated for a wide variety of conditions, such as osteoarthritis, fibromyalgia, migraines, tennis elbow, knee and back injuries, carpal tunnel syndrome, and whiplash. Dr. Ross Hauser, a medical doctor specializing in physical medicine and rehabilitation and one of the leading experts in the field of prolotherapy, unravels the mystery surrounding this unusual procedure in his book, *Prolo Your Pain Away!*

The kind of pain prolotherapy treats is musculoskeletal, involving both your muscles and bones. It is caused, Hauser says, by weak or damaged tissue that no longer holds your bones together properly. Either the bones rub against each other, or the neighboring muscles work too hard trying to keep things connected. That hurts — sometimes not only in the spot where the tendons and ligaments are weak, but down your leg, across your shoulders, or into your fingers. This is called ligament referred pain, pain that travels along certain patterns from an original source to other parts of your body.

If your doctor is unfamiliar with ligament referral pain patterns, he may not be able to pinpoint where your pain actually originates. That means you could be misdiagnosed, treated with the wrong medication, even undergo surgery — and still be in pain.

A prolotherapist, trained in these referral pain patterns, is able to attack the source of your pain. He injects the injured area with natural substances, and sometimes a small amount of an anesthetic, to alert your immune system that something is wrong. Blood and nutrients rush to the scene and get busy growing new, healthy tissue. The results are stronger, thicker ligaments that provide better support for your bones and joints.

The normal treatment routine runs for six weeks and begins with a thorough evaluation. You receive the injections, then give your body a chance to heal. At the end of the sixth week, your prolotherapist re-evaluates your pain. "Four treatments are normally required to eliminate pain," says Hauser. "Because everyone is unique, some people may only require one treatment while others will require as many as eight treatments. Rarely are more needed."

If prolotherapy is so successful, why haven't you heard of it before? Maybe because the whole basis of the treatment is contrary to what most doctors, trainers, physical therapists, and chiropractors recommend. For soft tissue injuries, like sprains, you've always been told to fight the inflammation with rest, ice, compression, and elevation (RICE). But Hauser explains, "The short-term result of this treatment is a reduction in pain. However, the RICE treatment decreases blood flow, preventing immune cells from getting to the injured area. This impairs the healing process, causes greater pain long-term, and increases the chance of incomplete healing of the injured ligament."

He offers a different approach: movement, exercise, analgesic, and treatment (MEAT). "Movement and gentle range-of-motion exercises improve blood flow to the area. If movement of the joint is painful, then isometric exercises should be performed. Isometric exercising involves contracting a muscle without movement of the affected joint. An example of this is a handshake. Both parties squeeze, creating a muscle contraction without joint movement."

He recommends only natural pain relievers or pain relievers that don't decrease inflammation, like acetaminophen. NSAIDs (nonsteroidal anti-inflammatory drugs), like ibuprofen and aspirin, decrease swelling. "Swelling tells the body, especially the brain, that an area of the body has been injured. The immune system is activated to send immune cells to the injured area. In the case of a soft tissue injury, inflammation is the cure for the problem."

And last, he recommends treatments that increase blood flow and cell movement to the injured area, such as physical therapy, massage, chiropractic care, ultrasound, and electrical stimulation.

Using MEAT allows complete healing of the injury, Hauser says. Prolotherapy often is used after traditional treatments have left an area weak and painful.

Dr. C. Everett Koop, former U.S. Surgeon General, is among those who have found relief with prolotherapy. He was so impressed with his results, in fact, that he even became trained in giving treatments. He says an accurate diagnosis is essential, and the therapy must be done by someone trained in prolotherapy. But he warns that prolotherapy is not a cure-all for all pain.

To find a trained prolotherapist in your area, check the referral list in the back of Hauser's book or call the American Association of Orthopedic Medicine at 1-800-992-2063. There are fees for this information.

You can also request a state listing of prolotherapists by sending a self-addressed, stamped envelope to: American College of Osteopathic Pain Management & Sclerotherapy (ACOPMS), 303 S. Ingram Court, Middletown, DE 19709. Or call 1-800-471-6114.

To order a copy of *Prolo Your Pain Away!* from Beulah Land Press, call 1-800-797-7656.

Heal yourself with humor

"Patch Adams," a movie starring Robin Williams, is about an unusual doctor who uses humor to help his patients feel better. Even before the success of that movie, hospitals were beginning to embrace this aspect of healing. Some of them provide humor rooms or carts for their patients. Loma Linda University, where much research on the healing power of humor has taken place, has a "Laughter Library," with humorous items patients can check out.

Humor may indeed help you keep a positive attitude through difficult times, such as dealing with a serious illness. But research finds that humor and laughter may also help prevent you from getting sick and could even help you live longer.

According to David Weeks, author of *Eccentrics: A Study of Sanity and Strangeness* (Kodansha Globe 1996), eccentrics live 20 to 25 years longer than average. It's probably because these intelligent, creative people don't take themselves seriously and are frequently blessed with a great sense of humor.

Here are four ways laughter can make you healthier.

▶ **Gives your body a workout.** Laughter has been called jogging for your internal organs. Whenever you laugh, you breathe deeper, which puts more oxygen in your bloodstream, and your diaphragm contracts and relaxes. Your heart rate and blood pressure also increase when you laugh, like it does when you exercise. However, after laughing, your heart rate and blood pressure decrease to lower levels than before you laughed. Dr. William Fry, a researcher specializing in the physical effects of laughter on your body, says that 20 seconds of a good "belly laugh" benefits your heart as much as three minutes of hard rowing.

▶ **Boosts your immune system.** Studies find that laughter can increase the activity of your immune system, which could help you fight disease. Dr. Lee Burk of Loma Linda University found that laughter increases several measurements of immune system activity, including natural killer cells, which attack virus and tumor cells; immunoglobulin A, which protects the upper respiratory tract; gamma interferon, which helps activate different parts of your immune system; and T cells, which are a specific type of white blood cell.

▶ **Eases stress.** When you're stressed out, a good laugh always makes you feel better. Research confirms that laughter actually reduces your body's production of cortisol and other stress-related hormones. An excess of these hormones in your body can be harmful, contributing to heart disease, cancer, depression, osteoporosis, and loss of brain function.

▶ **Chases away anger.** Have you ever been so angry you thought you were going to burst, and then something funny happened and you burst into laughter instead? It's difficult to laugh and be angry at the same time. So the next time someone cuts you off in traffic, instead of shaking your fist at them, just laugh. You'll feel better, and you may live longer. Remember, he who laughs — lasts.

Discover the healing power of magnets

When Michelle Wendall's horse began limping, a friend loaned her an odd contraption to strap onto his leg. It contained magnets, she said, and it would help relieve the pain in his knee without medication. "I thought it was crazy at first," Michelle admitted. "But it was worth a try to keep from paying another vet bill. Within days, he was running and jumping like he was 10 years younger. I was amazed."

The magnets were so successful on her horse, Michelle wondered if they might help relieve her husband's back pain. She did some research and discovered that the use of therapeutic magnets is growing rapidly. They are used and endorsed by professional athletes and celebrities, including Hank Aaron, Dan Marino, and golfer Bob Murphy.

The field of therapeutic magnets is also becoming a big-money industry. One of the leading producers, a Japanese company called Nikken, has gross sales of over $10 billion. The devices can cost anywhere from a few dollars to more than $1,000.

Despite all the hype, scientific evidence to support the healing power of magnets has been skimpy. The Food and Drug Administration hasn't approved the use of magnets, but it hasn't banned them either. Although much of the scientific community is skeptical about magnets, clinical research on the subject is just beginning, and early results look promising.

At Baylor College of Medicine in Houston, Dr. Carlos Vallbona and his colleagues tested magnets on 50 people with post-polio syndrome. They treated 29 people with magnets, while the rest of the volunteers wore fake magnets on their painful areas. Pain decreased in 76 percent of the people treated with real magnets, while only 19 percent of the people treated with fake magnets reported pain relief.

No one knows for sure why magnets might work. Some scientists think they act on iron particles in your blood or interact with your body's electrical system to stimulate better blood flow. Others believe magnetic fields trigger the healing action of your cells at a molecular level, interfere with your perception of pain, or stimulate the release of pain-relieving chemicals called endorphins.

If you decide to try magnets for your pain, don't just tape that strawberry-shaped magnet that's hanging on your refrigerator to your aching back. The strength of magnets is measured in gauss. The typical refrigerator magnet has about 60 gauss, while most therapeutic magnets have a strength of 300 to 4,000 gauss. The people in the Baylor study were treated with magnets of 300 to 500 gauss for 45-minutes.

Experts emphasize that more studies are needed to confirm whether magnets work to relieve pain. Although no side effects have been reported from the use of the devices, the possibility that there could be harmful side effects hasn't been ruled out.

Colds and Flu

9 ways to comfort coughs and colds

An occasional cold is a fact of life, but you don't have to take the sniffling, sneezing, coughing, and aching lying down. Here are nine ways to sidestep a cold or soothe the symptoms.

Soup it up. Chicken soup is ..e classic mother's remedy for colds and flu, and research shows that mom was right on the mark. One study found that even when chicken soup was diluted 200 times, it still interfered with the substances that trigger colds. Other studies found that hot soup can break up congestion and thin out mucous secretions.

Wash your hands. You don't have to catch every cold that comes along. Cold viruses are spread by touching infected respiratory secretions on someone's skin or on a surface, like a doorknob, and then touching your own eyes, nose, or mouth. You can also catch a cold by inhaling infectious particles in the air from a cough or sneeze. To reduce your chances of catching a cold, wash your hands frequently, and don't touch your eyes, nose, or mouth. Use soap and rub your hands together vigorously for best results. Plain soap works fine. The popular antibacterial soaps don't provide extra protection against colds because they only kill bacteria, not viruses.

Get steamed up. If a stuffy nose is making you miserable, jump in the shower. Hot, moist air can temporarily clear clogged nasal passages and help you breathe easier. A humidifier can also help. If you don't have one, you can make one. Just pour boiling water in a bowl, lean over it with a towel covering your head, and breathe deeply. Add some chamomile flowers to the water for extra relief. Chamomile helps clear clogged sinuses and soothes irritated throats.

Drink plenty of fluids. It's very important to get plenty of fluids when you have a cold or the flu, particularly if you have a fever. To prevent dehydration, and to thin the mucus in your lungs so you can cough it up, get at least eight to 10 cups of liquids a day.

Round up some vitamin C. Many people think vitamin C can prevent colds. While that hasn't been proven, studies have found that it may reduce the length of time you suffer cold symptoms. Taking supplements containing mega-doses of vitamin C isn't a good idea. Although too much vitamin C probably won't kill you, large doses may cause kidney stones, nausea, abdominal cramps, and diarrhea. To get vitamin C naturally, eat sweet red peppers, green peppers, citrus fruits, and strawberries.

Make a honey of a cough syrup. Drugstore shelves are crammed with cough syrups, but if you don't like taking medicine, you can make your own natural cough syrup. Mix the juice of one lemon with two tablespoons of glycerine and 12 teaspoons of honey. Take one teaspoon every half hour, stirring before each use. For another soothing and tasty cough reliever, combine 8 ounces of warm pineapple juice and two teaspoons of honey.

Go bananas. Bananas are delicious and loaded with folic acid, potassium, magnesium, and fiber, but did you know they may help quiet a cough? Heartburn is responsible for one in 10 chronic coughs. Research shows that eating bananas may bring relief from heartburn and the cough it causes.

Think zinc. Another nutrient that's controversial in the treatment of colds is zinc. Some studies have found that people with colds who use zinc gluconate lozenges recover from their colds more quickly than others. Other studies haven't shown any positive effects. If you want to try them, keep this in mind. Not only do they have a bad taste, they can cause nausea.

Make more friends. You can never have too many friends, right? A recent study found that having many social connections may make you less likely to catch a cold. The study found that people with six or more types of social ties — friend, spouse, parent, work mate, etc.

— were four times less likely to get a cold than those with three or fewer types of social connections. Researchers think extra psychological support or increased exposure to different viruses, which helps build immunity, could be the reason.

6 herbal remedies worth a try

Herbalists have their own tried-and-true remedies for coughs, colds, and the flu. Here are a few of the most popular.

▶ **Marshmallow root** *(Althaea officinalis).* When you have a cold, just the thought of sipping a warm cup of cocoa with fluffy marshmallows melting on top is probably enough to make you feel better. But did you know marshmallows were originally made from a plant, and this plant may help ease your cold symptoms? The dried root of the marshmallow plant contains 5 to 10 percent mucilage, which is a substance that becomes a tacky gel when mixed with liquid. Mucilage forms a protective layer over the membranes of your throat, reducing irritation and coughing. Marshmallow is usually taken as a tea or syrup. To make the tea, put one to two teaspoons of ground root in about 5 ounces of cold water. Allow it to sit for about an hour, then warm it and drink it.

▶ **Slippery elm** *(Ulmus fulva).* The inner bark of the slippery elm tree, also called the red elm or sweet elm, is a traditional remedy among Native Americans. They once used it to make a poultice for wounds and burns and to treat stomach problems. The mucilage in slippery elm soothes irritated throats and reduces coughing. You can drink it as a tea, or you can buy slippery elm lozenges. The Food and Drug Administration (FDA) says slippery elm is safe and effective, and it has no known side effects.

▶ **Mullein flower** *(Verbascum thapsus).* This plant has been used to treat a multitude of conditions from hemorrhoids to earaches. Its yellow flowers have even been used to make hair dye. This herb's most common use, however, is in the treatment of respiratory ailments. Mullein flowers contain mucilage. This soothes your throat and acts as a mild expectorant, loosening phlegm and mucus, which quiets your cough. To make a tea of mullein flowers, use three to four teaspoonfuls in about 5 ounces of water.

▶ **Licorice** *(Glycyrrhiza glabra).* The scientific name for licorice — glycyrrhiza — comes from the Greek words for "sweet roots." When you hear the word "licorice," you probably think of candy, but the therapeutic use of this plant dates back to the Roman Empire. It was used to treat coughs because it helps get rid of mucus. If you have high blood pressure, this is one herb to stay away from. Its active ingredient, glycyrrhizic acid, is similar to an adrenal hormone called aldosterone, and even small amounts can raise your blood pressure dangerously high.

▶ **Echinacea** *(Echinacea purpurea, Echinacea angustifolia).* When it comes to cold prevention, echinacea has the most established history of all the herbs. Also called the purple coneflower, this member of the daisy family grows in the Midwestern United States. It was used by Native Americans to treat colds, coughs, sore throats, toothaches, and even snakebites. Echinacea seems to fight colds and flu by boosting your immune system. In a recent study, the white blood cells of men who took an echinacea supplement for four days were three times more effective at killing bacteria.

▶ **Elderberry** *(Sambucus nigra).* The last time you had the flu, did you think you'd never get over it? Research shows that elderberries may make your next bout with the flu a little shorter. One study gave a standardized elderberry extract, called Sambucol, to people with the flu. Within two days, improvement — including fever reduction — was seen in over 90 percent of the people taking the elderberry extract. It took the people who didn't take the extract six days to show an improvement. Look for elderberry extract as an ingredient in commercial syrups and lozenges.

Superbugs — the latest threat to your health

While everyone seems to be working frantically to thwart the effects of the Y2K computer bug, superbugs of a different kind may be becoming more and more of a threat. Experts fear that someday strains of bacteria resistant to all known antibiotics may become the world's number one health problem. Ironically, it may be the overuse of the very antibiotics used to combat bacteria that might cause you to fall victim to these superbugs.

When antibiotics were discovered in the first part of the 20th century, they revolutionized the medical field. Suddenly, doctors were able to effectively combat deadly infections and save millions of lives. This was particularly significant during World War II. The death toll may have been much higher from infected wounds had it not been for antibiotics.

However, it wasn't long before antibiotics were being prescribed for less severe problems, often for conditions that wouldn't respond to antibiotics anyway. Antibiotics can only fight infections caused by bacteria. They are useless against infections caused by a virus. In 1992, doctors handed out about 12 million antibiotic prescriptions for colds, upper respiratory tract infections, and bronchitis. But since viruses cause about 90 percent of those conditions, antibiotics didn't help.

What they did do was contribute to developing resistant strains of bacteria. Whenever germs are exposed to antibiotics, most of them are killed, but if any remain, they can become immune to that antibiotic. Those resistant bacteria can then multiply rapidly — a group of bacteria can double in size within 20 minutes. That's why it's important to finish a prescription of antibiotics once you start taking them.

The medical community is becoming more aware of the magnitude of the antibiotic resistance problem, but many doctors are still prescribing unnecessary antibiotics. According to the Centers for Disease Control and Prevention (CDC), people consume 235 million doses of antibiotics yearly, and it is estimated that 20 percent to 50 percent of that use is not necessary.

Another factor that may be contributing to antibiotic resistance is the overuse of antibiotics in livestock. Most of the millions of pounds of antibiotics given to animals are intended to stimulate growth, not fight infections.

While you may not be able to do anything about the antibiotics given to animals, you can help fight antibiotic resistance by following a few guidelines.

- ▶ Don't ask your doctor to prescribe an antibiotic for a cold or the flu. Many doctors say they prescribe antibiotics because their patients expect it.

- ▶ If your doctor prescribes an antibiotic, ask questions. Make sure it is necessary for you to take that drug.

- ▶ Follow directions given by your doctor or pharmacist exactly. Take your medicine at the proper time and finish the entire prescription. Don't stop taking it just because you feel better. Some bacteria may still be alive.

- ▶ Always wash your hands thoroughly and handle food properly to prevent spreading bacteria in the first place.

- ▶ Never save medication to give to someone else later.

Colon Cancer

Go vegetarian to ward off colon cancer

Have you always thought a meal wasn't a meal without meat? If so, you may be increasing your risk of colon cancer. Numerous studies have found that eating red meat boosts your risk. Now new evidence shows eating white meat, like fish and chicken, may also raise your risk.

A study of Seventh Day Adventists in California examined the link between diet and colon cancer. Researchers found that eating meat was the strongest dietary risk factor. People who ate either red or white meat more than four times a week were two to three times as likely to develop colon cancer as those who never ate meat. The study also found that legumes, like peas and beans, can protect you from colon cancer.

Vegetarian may be the way to go if you're concerned about colon cancer. A healthy vegetarian diet includes a variety of plant-based foods, including grains and legumes.

Scientists at Cornell University recently developed a vegetarian diet pyramid, similar to the traditional food pyramid. As its basis, it recommends a wide variety of plant foods — fruits and vegetables, whole grains, and legumes. The next level includes nuts, seeds, dairy products or soy milk, and plant oils. Optional items include eggs, sweets, and alcohol to be consumed in small amounts.

The chart also emphasizes daily physical exercise and plenty of water, two things that are important to any healthy eating plan.

If you are one of the estimated 14 million Americans who consider themselves vegetarians, following this diet pyramid is a good way to make sure you're getting the proper nutrients.

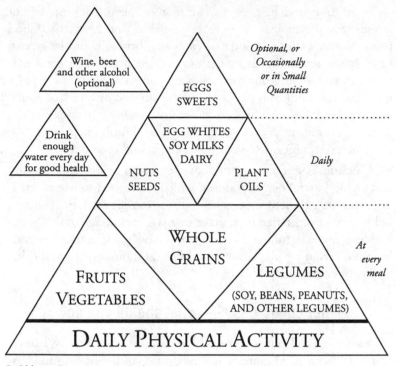

Wine, beer and other alcohol (optional)

Drink enough water every day for good health

EGGS
SWEETS

Optional, or Occasionally or in Small Quantities

EGG WHITES
SOY MILKS
DAIRY

NUTS
SEEDS

PLANT
OILS

Daily

WHOLE
GRAINS

LEGUMES

FRUITS
VEGETABLES

(SOY, BEANS, PEANUTS, AND OTHER LEGUMES)

At every meal

DAILY PHYSICAL ACTIVITY

If you want to try eating vegetarian, plan your meals carefully. If you don't, you could become deficient in the following nutrients:

Vitamin B12. This vitamin can only be found in foods of animal origin. If you eat dairy products every day, you're probably getting enough. If you are a strict vegetarian and don't eat any animal foods, you could be deficient. Ask your doctor if you need vitamin B12 supplements.

Vitamin D. Sunlight and fortified dairy products are the main sources of vitamin D for most people. If you don't get out in the sun much or eat dairy products, you might need supplements. Since vitamin D is the most toxic of all vitamins, don't overdo it. Taking too much can cause headache, nausea, diarrhea, kidney damage, and heart disease.

Iron. An iron deficiency is a common problem that's usually not serious. Symptoms include fatigue, pale skin, and headache. Good plant sources of iron include dried beans, broccoli, turnip greens, dried fruits, sesame seeds, and iron-fortified breads and cereals. If you're careful about your food choices, you shouldn't need supplements. If you think you do, check with your doctor first. Too much iron can be dangerous. Symptoms of iron overload include nausea, diarrhea, vomiting blood, pale skin, and bluish nails and lips. Extreme cases can cause convulsions, coma, and even death.

Calcium. A recent study of people at risk for colon cancer found that eating low-fat dairy products, which are a good source of calcium, may actually return precancerous colon cells to normal. If you follow a strict vegetarian diet, make sure you get enough of this bone-building mineral from other sources. Good plant sources include broccoli, turnip greens, beans, dried figs, sunflower seeds, and calcium-fortified cereals and juices.

Fiber controversy — what should you do?

Your mom called it roughage. Nutritionists call it fiber. Whatever you call it, you need more of it. Numerous studies have found that fiber may protect you from constipation, hemorrhoids, diabetes, obesity, heart disease, and colon cancer.

The Food and Drug Administration (FDA) even allows products high in fiber to make health claims on their labels.

But now a new study has cast doubt on the protective effect of fiber against colon cancer. The researchers used information from over 88,000 nurses and came to the conclusion that eating high-fiber foods had no effect on colon cancer risk.

Scientists are trying to determine why this study had different results from many other studies. They are not sure if it's fiber that protects against colon cancer or something else in a high-fiber diet.

One reason fiber may protect against colon cancer is because it prevents constipation. Studies have found that people who are frequently constipated have a greater risk of developing colon cancer.

The type of fiber you consume could also be the key. In one study, people who got their fiber from vegetables had a 43 percent reduced risk of colon cancer. Fiber from fruit had a smaller protective effect, and grain fiber had no protective effect.

For now, the bulk of evidence shows eating a high-fiber diet helps prevent colon cancer. A recent review of 19 studies on the effect of grain fiber on colon cancer revealed that 16 of the studies found a protective effect, while the other three showed no effect.

No one is suggesting you eat less fiber. In fact, the National Cancer Institute says you need to eat more. They recommend 20 to 30 grams a day, instead of the 11 grams most people take in daily.

To avoid side effects, such as excessive gas, add fiber to your diet gradually, and don't get more than 35 grams a day.

Squelch colon cancer with supplements

Perhaps you got your blue eyes from your mother, and your curly hair from your father. Along with all those innocent genes, you may have inherited the gene for colon cancer. Approximately 20 percent of the people diagnosed with colon cancer have a family history of the disease. Luckily, taking vitamin and mineral supplements may keep that genetic predisposition from turning deadly.

Folic acid. This B-vitamin has been in the news lately because it helps protect against heart and artery disease. It does this by limiting the amount of a substance called homocysteine in your blood. New evidence suggests it may also protect against cancer. Folic acid works with vitamin B12 to convert homocysteine to methionine, an amino acid. Methionine helps maintain the genes that keep your cells from becoming cancerous. This means a shortage of folic acid and vitamin B12 might increase your risk of cancer.

Studies support the idea that folic acid may reduce the risk of developing colon cancer. In one large study involving over 88,000 nurses, women who took multivitamins containing folic acid for more than 15 years were 75 percent less likely to develop colon cancer than women who didn't use supplements. Women who took the supplements for between five to 14 years were about 20 percent less likely to develop it.

Calcium. You know calcium is good for your bones, but new research indicates it's also good for your intestines. Results of a four-year study show that calcium supplements reduce the risk of recurring colon polyps. Called large bowel adenomas, these polyps are not cancerous but can become cancerous. If you've had one, you're likely to develop more. Researchers gave the people with a history of polyps a 1,200 milligram (mg) calcium supplement or a placebo. The people who got the calcium supplements had a 19 percent reduction in recurrence of one polyp and a 24 percent decrease in total number of polyps.

Vitamin E. Vitamin E is a powerful antioxidant that may protect against colon cancer. A study of over 800 men and women found that people who took vitamin E supplements over a 10-year period had a 57 percent lower risk of developing colon cancer. The average amount of vitamin E taken by people in the study was 200 international units (IU) daily.

How to enhance garlic's benefits

Every time you make spaghetti for your family, you could be protecting them from cancer — if you add garlic to your sauce. Numerous studies have found that garlic may protect against several kinds of cancer.

Garlic has a complex chemical structure. It's composed of over 100 chemical parts. Scientists have pinpointed those most likely to protect against cancer — diallyl trisulfides and diallyl disulfides. Animal studies have found that these compounds may protect against cancers of the lung, colon, kidney, mouth, skin, and breast.

Several studies on humans have also supported garlic's cancer-fighting benefits. One study found that men who ate garlic or took garlic supplements at least twice a week were less likely to develop prostate cancer. In another study, people who ate the most garlic were less likely to get colorectal cancer than those who ate less garlic. A recent analysis of several studies found that eating just one clove of garlic a day protected against stomach and colon cancers, but garlic supplements had no effect.

If you want to take advantage of garlic's cancer protection, it's important how you prepare it. A recent study found that heating garlic just after it's crushed causes it to lose some of its cancer-fighting abilities.

Researchers gave rats corn oil either with or without garlic. The rats given crushed garlic that was allowed to "rest" at room temperature for 10 minutes and then heated in a microwave oven showed a 41 percent reduction in cell changes linked to cancer. Garlic that was allowed to rest and then roasted in a conventional oven resulted in a 21 percent reduction in cancerous cell changes. But garlic that was heated immediately after crushing had no anti-cancer effect.

Crushing or chopping garlic releases an enzyme that is present in some garlic cells. This allows it to come into contact with and activate the compounds that help protect against cancer. If the garlic is heated immediately after chopping, the enzyme is destroyed before it has time to act on the compounds and convert them.

In the study, raw garlic had the greatest cancer-fighting effect. If you can't stand the thought of biting into a raw clove of garlic, just let it rest before cooking. Then you can take advantage of its aroma, as well as its cancer protection.

Fight cancer with exotic Indian spice

If you're a regular at the Indian restaurant in your neighborhood, you may be protecting yourself from cancer. Turmeric, a spice used in Indian cooking, contains a substance called curcumin, which gives turmeric its yellow color. Turmeric is found in yellow rice, and it's the main ingredient in curry.

Numerous studies find that curcumin may help prevent cancers of the colon, breast, stomach, lung, liver, blood, skin, and mouth. More research is needed to confirm its cancer-fighting abilities, but if you like the flavor of turmeric, eat plenty of it. You could be warding off cancer.

Inexpensive way to prevent colon cancer

Aspirin is a blessing to headache sufferers, but relieving pain is just the beginning of the things this simple little pill can do.

Studies have found that aspirin can help prevent heart attacks and strokes by helping your blood flow more smoothly. It may also help prevent Alzheimer's disease by reducing inflammation in the brain that could cause brain cell damage. And it may help prevent several types of cancer, particularly colorectal cancer.

One large study found that taking a daily aspirin for 20 years cut the risk of colorectal cancer almost in half.

However, a recent 12-year study, the Physician's Health Study, found that aspirin had no effect on risk. Researchers think the dosage and the length of treatment period in the Physician's Health Study could have contributed to those negative findings.

Another large study, the Women's Health Study, is underway now, and researchers hope it will provide more information.

In the meantime, a test tube study has found that aspirin may prevent genetic mutations that lead to a particular type of colon cancer. Researchers studied a severe, inherited kind of cancer called "hereditary nonpolyposis colorectal cancer," or HNPCC. This type of cancer runs in families, usually affecting three or more close relatives. In test tubes, aspirin caused unstable cells to commit suicide instead of mutating and becoming tumors.

Even if colorectal cancer runs in your family, talk with your doctor before taking daily aspirin. Aspirin can cause side effects, like stomach problems, and sometimes interacts with other medications, particularly blood thinners.

Constipation

Natural ways to keep things moving

When it comes to regulating the natural rhythms of your body, the fewer drugs you use, the better.

Several years ago, the FDA proposed a ban on phenolphthalein, the active ingredient in many laxatives. Researchers said it was a potential cancer risk for people who use it for long periods of time or at higher than normal doses.

If you've relied on laxatives in the past, now is the time to try natural ways to keep your plumbing on a regular schedule.

Fill up on fiber. Not getting enough fiber in your diet is the most common cause of constipation. Vegetables, fruits, whole grains, and legumes are good sources of fiber.

Drink plenty of water. Drink six to eight cups of water every day. Water helps soften your stools so you can pass them more easily.

Check out the latest buzz. A small study confirmed the age-old remedy of drinking a mixture of one to three tablespoons of honey and water to get the bowels moving. But if you have irritable bowel syndrome, it could make your symptoms worse.

Try a taste of the islands. Studies have shown that bromelain, an enzyme found in fresh, frozen, or canned pineapple, helps with regularity. Although most of the bromelain is in the pineapple's stem, some nutritionists say eating just 4 ounces of pineapple a day will help relieve constipation.

Mix in some psyllium. Psyllium is a powder form of vegetable fiber that is widely available in products such as Metamucil. This helps gather your waste in bulk and eases the removal process.

Have some fun. Exercising regularly can keep your bowels in good working order. A mild workout often stimulates movement of the bowels and puts an end to your discomfort.

Beware of side effects. Common medications, such as sedatives, aluminum or calcium antacids, diuretics, iron supplements, antidepressants, and cough syrup with codeine, can cause constipation. If you think a drug you're taking is causing your constipation, talk with your doctor. But don't stop taking it without his approval.

═══════════

The versatility of pineapple

Bromelain, the same pineapple enzyme that helps you stay regular, also shows promise blocking E. coli, the bacteria responsible for travelers' diarrhea.

In a recent study, a dose of bromelain kept more than half of the piglets exposed to E. coli from developing diarrhea. Among those piglets who were not treated with bromelain, none escaped diarrhea. In fact, the more of the enzyme a piglet was given, the better his chances got.

Although the bromelain enzyme is present throughout the pineapple, its concentration is much higher in the stem of the plant than in the fruit. Eating pineapple chunks probably isn't going to pack a strong enough bromelain punch to beat back E. coli. Fortunately, bromelain is available in over-the-counter tablet form.

The next time you're off to some exotic port of call, remember the versatility of your favorite exotic fruit.

═══════════

Depression

4 natural ways to ditch depression

Let's face it. Most people get the blues every once in a while. The good news is a long-term study of depression has revealed new ways to treat it without dangerous drugs.

Get physical. Exercise gets you out of the house, encourages you to interact with others and meet new people, and gets your mind off your problems. Numerous studies show that people who get regular exercise are less likely to become depressed than people who don't. Exercise actually stimulates the production of dopamine and serotonin, chemicals in your brain that lift your spirits.

In fact, some studies have shown that exercising regularly is just as effective at treating depression as taking antidepressants and getting counseling. In almost all cases, when people added an exercise program to their drug or counseling treatment, their conditions improved more rapidly and significantly.

Consider herbal remedies. More and more people are using herbs to treat depression. If you want to try herbal remedies, ask your doctor for advice. But don't stop taking medicine he has prescribed without his approval.

▶ **St John's wort.** Studies have proven that this herbal antidepressant works well for many people. This is great news because herbal supplements have fewer and less severe side effects than most antidepressants. Although St. John's wort relieves mild to moderate depression, it doesn't relieve severe depression, manic-depression, or obsessive-compulsive disorder.

▶ **Kava.** This tropical-sounding herb is another popular mood enhancer. Kava, sometimes called kava kava, comes from the South Pacific and has been soothing islanders for generations.

It's been shown to improve mood, reduce anxiety, and raise mental alertness. However, some experts are concerned about a link between kava and toxic liver disease. Talk to your doctor before taking kava and have him monitor your treatment.

► **Valerian.** This herb aids sleep and calms anxiety. As with other herbal treatments, valerian works slowly so it might take more time to see results than with traditional medications.

Keep a song in your heart. It is said music tames the savage beast, but can it do the same for your savage mood? Many mental health professionals seem to think it can. Research shows that relaxing and finding distractions from your problems will keep you in better spirits than if you dwell on them. Those who talk about their frustrations tend to become more negative. Music, art, and other mellow distractions are just the trick for fending off life's daily annoyances that threaten to overwhelm you.

Kick an unhealthy habit. As if you needed another reason not to smoke, depression and tobacco use have been closely linked. One study showed that heavy smokers were almost twice as likely to develop severe depression as people who smoked infrequently. Don't let tobacco bring you down — kick the habit.

Surprising cause of depression

Is it possible to "catch" depression just like you might catch a cold? Some disturbing findings suggest it might be. German researchers say a virus that causes severe depression in horses, cows, sheep, and cats has now been found in humans. This virus, called the Borna virus, was first identified in horses in the late 1800s.

Scientists aren't sure how the virus causes depression, but it seems to interfere with the normal functioning of the part of the brain that controls emotions.

Many people infected with the Borna virus have shown improvement after being treated with anti-viral medication or antidepressants.

If you're worried about eating meat from infected animals, don't be. Experts say the virus isn't transmitted that way, but they're still wondering if it can "jump" from animals to people.

Change your mood with these foods

You are what you eat. If you want to chase away the blues, look at what you're eating. Studies confirm that certain foods can help beat depression.

Perk up and smile. If you don't feel like yourself until after your first cup of coffee, you're not alone. Many people say caffeine keeps them alert and improves their mood. Now medical evidence is starting to back this up.

In a 10-year study of female nurses, caffeine seemed to make a big difference in the rate of serious depression. Women who were regular coffee drinkers had lower rates of suicide than women who didn't drink coffee.

Caffeine is the most widely used stimulant in the world, and about 75 percent of it is consumed from coffee. While you shouldn't deal with depression by drinking four pots of coffee every morning, how much or how little caffeine you get could be affecting the way you look at the world.

Warm up to a wholesome breakfast. What has the power to fill your stomach and warm your soul at the same time? Nothing more extravagant than old, reliable oatmeal. Researchers have learned that complex carbohydrates, found in vegetables, fruits, and grains like oats, can trigger the production of serotonin. Raising the levels of serotonin in your brain can raise your spirits. The increase brought on by just one bowl of oatmeal can improve your mood for several hours.

Enjoy a glass of milk. Doctors have found a direct link between depression and low levels of protein in the diet. In one study, not only did depression increase as patients stuck to a low-protein diet, but their lifestyle and quality of life also declined.

Most people get more than enough protein, but if you don't, add some meat and dairy products to your diet. Vegetables and grains also contain protein but in lesser amounts.

Go fish. Omega-3 fatty acids, powerful weapons in the fight against heart disease, may also help you win the battle against depression. Research shows that in countries where people eat a lot of fish, a good source of omega-3s, the incidence of depression is low. In one study, Japanese students who took a daily fish oil supplement for three months were less hostile and aggressive than their peers.

Some experts warn that there are too many other cultural differences to be absolutely sure fish are helping to ward off depression. In the meantime, eating more fish can't hurt. At the very least, you'll be giving your heart a treat, and that's enough to make anybody smile.

Raising grandchildren could cause depression

Today, more and more grandparents are taking on the responsibility of raising their grandchildren. And for some, the stress might be too much.

A recent study from the National Survey of Families and Households determined that seniors who were the primary caregivers for their grandchildren were almost twice as likely to suffer from depression than those who weren't.

Among the caregivers, a higher income and older age seemed to lower the risk of depression. The same goes for marriage and good overall health. These facts are making experts wonder what is really causing the depression. Is it the children or the circumstances that caused the grandparents to become caregivers in the first place?

Escape depression and arthritis with natural supplement

Don't take depression lightly. It can be much more serious than just a temporary case of "the blues." Suicide is the eighth leading cause of death in the United States. In the 25 to 44 age group, it is the fourth leading cause of death, and it ranks third as the cause of death in people ages 15 to 24.

It's not surprising that antidepressant medication accounts for billions of dollars in sales every year. But these drugs are expensive, require a prescription, and can cause undesirable side effects, including sexual problems. It's also not surprising that people are constantly searching for new weapons to fight depression.

A natural supplement called S-adenosyl-methionine, or SAMe (pronounced "sammy"), recently appeared in stores in the United States. SAMe has been used in Europe for the last 20 years to treat depression and arthritis.

Studies find that SAMe is effective in treating about 70 percent of depressed people. This is about the same percentage as other treatments for depression, but it doesn't cause the side effects associated with most prescription antidepressants. It also usually works more quickly.

Volunteers in early studies who suffered with depression and arthritis reported that their joint pain was lessened while taking SAMe. Later studies found that people with arthritis got as much pain relief from SAMe as they did from taking NSAIDs, like ibuprofen.

Exactly what is this miraculous substance that can improve your mood and your joints? It's a compound your body makes from methionine, an amino acid. It works by donating part of itself, a methyl group, to your tissues and organs. The chain of events this donation sets in motion help maintain cell membranes, remove toxic substances from your body, and help produce neurotransmitters, like serotonin and dopamine. It is the enhanced production of neurotransmitters that accounts for SAMe's antidepressive effect.

After SAMe donates its methyl group, the process of breaking down what is left also benefits your body. This breakdown creates other molecules, including sulfates. These sulfates, which help maintain healthy cartilage in your joints, account for how SAMe helps treat arthritis.

So far, SAMe seems safe and effective, but it needs help from vitamin B12 and folic acid to work properly. If you decide to try SAMe, make sure you're getting enough of those vitamins.

These drugs can steal sexual desire

Anti-anxiety drugs

Generic name	Brand name
alprazolam	Xanax
chlordiazepoxide	Librium, Libritabs
diazepam	Valium, Valrelease
oxazepam	Serax

Antidepressants

Generic name	Brand name
amitriptyline hydrochloride	Elavil
amoxapine	Asendin
citalopram hydrobromide	Celexa
clomipramine hydrochloride	Anafranil
desipramine hydrochloride	Norpramin
doxepin hydrochloride	Sinequan
fluoxetine hydrochloride	Prozac
imipramine hydrochloride	Tofranil
nortriptyline hydrochloride	Pamelor
paroxetine hydrochloride	Paxil
phenelzine sulfate	Nardil
protriptyline hydrochloride	Vivactil
sertraline hydrochloride	Zoloft
trazodone hydrochloride	Desyrel

Never stop taking a prescription drug without talking to your doctor first.

Diabetes

Preventing the silent killer

A sore on your leg that refuses to heal, bleeding gums, or a recurring bladder infection. They may seem harmless, but these symptoms should set alarm bells ringing. They could mean you're one of more than 16 million people in the United States with non-insulin dependent diabetes mellitus (NIDDM), more commonly known as Type 2 diabetes.

This deadly disease is reaching epidemic proportions, but because it can remain hidden for years, lurking behind damaged kidneys, nerves, or vision, one-third of those afflicted don't know they have it until it's too late.

The tragedy is that Type 2 diabetes cannot only be controlled but prevented — simply by making changes in your lifestyle. By combining the right diet and regular exercise, you can almost half your risk of developing diabetes.

Know the danger signs. Type 1 diabetes occurs in children or young adults whose bodies can't make the insulin they need to control their blood sugar levels. Type 2 is more likely to appear in adults over age 40 who can't make enough insulin or have problems using their insulin. Up to 95 percent of all diabetics fall into this second category. Your chances of joining them are greater if you:

► are overweight

► eat a high-fat diet

► do not exercise regularly

► have a family history of diabetes

► are African-American, Hispanic-American, Asian or Pacific Islander, or Native American

▶ had gestational diabetes (a temporary condition in pregnancy)

▶ have low levels of HDL cholesterol or high triglyceride levels

If you match up with two or more risk factors, you are a likely candidate for developing Type 2 diabetes.

Don't wait to lose weight. Even if you have inherited a tendency toward diabetes, you usually need a trigger, like obesity, to develop it. Just look at the statistics — 80 percent of all diabetics are overweight. Obesity has become the single most important cause of Type 2 diabetes.

The definition of obese is being 20 percent over your recommended weight. And if you carry those extra pounds around your middle, you're in more danger of developing this disease than if you are "pear-shaped."

Talk to your doctor about a safe and gradual weight-loss program that combines good nutrition and exercise.

Cheat diabetes with good nutrition. The American Diabetic Association recommends a sensible diet of fresh fruits and vegetables, complex carbohydrates, lean meat, and fish. Stay away from sugar, saturated fat, and high-cholesterol foods, and eat several small meals throughout the day. Although these guidelines apply to diabetics, they are also appropriate if you want to avoid this disease. Focus on getting these nutrients into your diet:

▶ **Fiber.** Many experts believe soluble fiber, like that found in whole grains, fruits, and vegetables, is your best bet for controlling your glucose levels and weight. Researchers at Harvard recently found that women who eat a diet high in fiber and low in sugar are much less likely to develop diabetes.

▶ **Chromium.** It helps insulin move glucose out of your blood stream and into your cells. If you are at risk for diabetes, get a healthy amount of chromium through foods like beef, liver, seafood, mushrooms, whole grains, asparagus, and nuts.

▶ **Magnesium.** Low levels can increase your risk of becoming insulin resistant. To keep your magnesium on track, eat beans, broccoli, corn, shellfish, and skim milk.

▶ **Zinc.** Studies show that if you lack zinc, you may have problems keeping your blood sugar level normal after eating. A survey found that only 6 percent of diabetics were getting their recommended daily allowance of zinc. That means supplementing might be good insurance against diabetes. Red meat, shellfish, and lima beans are your best bets to get more zinc naturally.

▶ **Vitamin A.** It plays a vital role in insulin control. The more effective your insulin is at controlling blood sugar, the less likely you are to develop diabetes. For a healthy dose of A, load up on richly colored fruits and vegetables like sweet potatoes, carrots, and spinach.

▶ **Vitamin E.** Researchers have found that low levels of vitamin E increase your risk of developing diabetes. In fact, one study found that men with low vitamin E levels were four times more likely to develop this disease. Vegetable oils such as safflower, canola, and corn oils; wheat germ; sunflower seeds; sweet potatoes; and shrimp are good sources of vitamin E.

▶ **Biotin.** A relatively unknown B vitamin, it may reduce the amount of insulin your body needs. You can get biotin naturally from liver, egg yolks, and cereals.

Work out for winning health. If you lead a fairly inactive life, your risk of developing diabetes is four times greater than if you exercise, say researchers at the Cooper Institute for Aerobics Research in Dallas, Texas. That makes exercise your most powerful weapon for preventing this disease and the one factor over which you have the most control. A brisk 20-minute walk three or four times a week is a small effort that can bring big results.

Reverse your diabetes

Would you believe that losing as little as five pounds can help reverse Type 2 diabetes? It's true, according to a study at the University of Texas Health Sciences Center in San Antonio.

Researchers followed more than 3,500 diabetics from the San Antonio Heart Study. After eight years, they found that 12 percent became non-diabetic. Although the disease technically can't be cured, eliminating the symptoms, even for a short time, is certainly a goal to strive for.

The factors that helped people reverse their diabetes included losing five pounds or more; increasing their HDL or "good" cholesterol; and lowering their blood glucose, triglycerides, and fasting insulin levels. Researchers found that it also helps if you're in a high socioeconomic group and develop diabetes at an older age.

The sooner your diabetes is detected, the easier it will be to avoid complications and possibly even reverse the disease. So pay attention to risk factors and symptoms, and see your doctor at the first sign of trouble.

New research says cut your carbohydrates

Can you give up French bread, pasta, baked potatoes, and your favorite fruit cobbler? If so, you may be able to control your blood sugar level without insulin or other medications, researchers say.

This radically different diet is still being tested, but a recent study showed that eating fewer carbohydrates may improve your glucose levels, help you lose weight, and even lower your blood pressure.

The study by the Sansum Medical Research Foundation in California found that Type 2 diabetics improved significantly when carbohydrates made up only 25 percent of their daily calories. When placed on a 55-percent carbohydrate diet, their blood sugar control worsened.

This research contradicts the American Diabetic Association's recommendation that your diet contain a 60-to-70-percent combination of carbohydrates and monounsaturated fats. Several years ago, the ADA revised its diet plan to include more, not fewer, carbohydrates.

Talk to your doctor before you make any changes as drastic as this new research proposes. What you eat and when you eat it are critical decisions for a diabetic. Just keep an ear out for further news on this controversial diet plan.

Fat: future fix for diabetes?

Eat a cheeseburger and prevent diabetes? Not quite, but researchers hope a polyunsaturated fat in certain foods may provide a new way to conquer this widespread disease.

Conjugated linoleic acid, or CLA, is a common fatty acid found mostly in red meat and cheese, and in small amounts in milk, eggs, chicken, yogurt, and cooking oil.

When CLA was isolated out of whole foods and tested on laboratory animals, it seemed to prevent Type 2 diabetes just as well as a certain group of diabetes-fighting drugs, the thiazolidinediones (TZDs). Researchers think it may someday become the first choice for prevention, since CLA actually reduces body fat. Traditional diabetes drugs often make you gain weight.

Although you can find CLA as a dietary supplement in many health stores, experts don't recommend rushing off to buy it. Instead, they advise getting CLA through whole foods. Several universities are trying to increase the CLA quality of different foods so you'll get more of it naturally.

"Here at Washington Sate University, we're working on enhancing a lot of dairy products," says Louise Peck, assistant professor of foods and nutrition. "Hopefully, we'll be able to enhance the natural CLA in some of these products and come up with something we can use instead of supplements."

Peck is quick to point out that there's a lot they still don't know about CLA. "We don't know the dosage that is going to be effective. We're just starting a study to determine that," she says. There are also concerns about possible liver damage and unknown side effects. But it is something that looks promising for the future, she concludes.

Heel to toe foot care for diabetics

One out of every 170 diabetics will have a foot amputated due to the nerve disorder peripheral neuropathy. Horrifying statistics considering you can prevent this tragic outcome with good foot care.

About a third of all diabetics suffer from neuropathy, which can cause special problems for your feet. Because this disorder damages your nerves, you may not feel pain from injuries or irritations. You are more likely to develop ulcers or infections, and your foot shape can actually change. So it's critical that you pay special attention to your shoes and feet.

The first step to better foot care is scheduling a thorough foot exam with your doctor at least once a year. However, if a problem arises between visits, don't wait — see your doctor right away. Whether you see a general practitioner, a diabetes specialist, or a podiatrist, make sure he tests the nerve function and circulation in your feet.

He should also check your skin and nails and take care of any routine maintenance you can't manage yourself. Talk about changes you've noticed. Do your feet feel different? Are they a different shape or color?

Then, each day, do everything you can to prevent a minor problem from becoming a major pain.

Examine your feet every day. Look for blisters, cuts, scrapes, sores, redness, bruises, infections, swelling, or bumps. Get someone to help you, or use a mirror if you can't see the bottoms of your feet.

Wash with mild soap. Use warm water (check the temperature with your wrist) and don't soak — that removes calluses that can protect sensitive spots. Dry them carefully, especially between your toes.

Treat dry skin. If your feet seem especially dry, check with your doctor to make sure you don't have athlete's foot, which needs special care. If it's just dry skin, apply a small amount of petroleum jelly or lotion before you put on your socks and shoes. (Most people don't need expensive specialty products.) This will keep your skin from cracking. But avoid moisturizing the skin between your toes.

Sock it to 'em. Wear socks that are soft and thick enough for extra protection. Choose material that will draw moisture away from your skin, like acrylic. Avoid cotton, which stays wet; thin, slippery socks or stockings; and any that have holes or seams.

Choose shoes with care. They should fit well even over your thickest socks, with enough room so your toes don't rub. Take any inserts with you when you go shopping to ensure a fool-proof fit. Don't assume you take the same size you've worn for years since your foot may become wider and flatter with the disease. If necessary, visit a pedorthist, a corrective shoe specialist.

In most cases, Medicare will pay for part of the cost of therapeutic shoes. To qualify, you must meet certain guidelines and have formal proof from your doctor.

Look before you lace. Before putting on your shoes, check inside for pebbles or other objects, and make sure your shoes don't have holes or tears that could cause injury.

Never go barefoot outside. Even indoors you need to be careful. Keep slippers by your bed to avoid bumping into things at night.

Take special care of your toenails. Cut them straight across, but file down sharp corners that might cut the next toe. If you develop a nail fungal infection, don't use an over-the-counter remedy without talking to your doctor first. Many oral medications work better.

Smooth out the rough spots. Use a dry towel or pumice stone to rub away dead skin.

Stay away from self-surgery. Don't cut off corns, calluses, or warts yourself, and never use nonprescription remedies to remove them. The harsh chemicals can damage the surrounding healthy tissue. Take these problems to your doctor.

Sleep tight tonight. Don't use hot water bottles or heating pads to warm your feet at night. Wear socks instead. If the bedcovers are especially irritating or heavy on your feet, buy a special hoop device from a medical supply store that holds the sheet off your legs.

Get your blood moving. Try not to cross your legs when you sit. This keeps the blood from flowing freely to your legs and feet.

Exercise will also improve circulation and may help take your mind off the pain.

———————

Cow protein may spell de'feet' for foot ulcers

If you're diabetic, finding a sore on your foot or leg may strike fear in your heart. After all, more than 56,000 diabetics have a limb amputated every year, usually due to an ulcer that refused to heal. That's why most doctors will consider any new treatment to reduce these shocking statistics — even one from the farm.

Bovine collagen is the latest remedy promising faster and more successful healing of diabetic sores. Even though it's still considered experimental, many experts are raving about how successful it's been. Dr. Lawrence Kollenberg, Director of the Garland County Foot Clinic in Arkansas, uses it and has cut his rate of amputation by about 94 percent.

Collagen is a natural protein found in the connective tissue of skin, bones, ligaments, and cartilage. It speeds up clotting so that the wound is more quickly sealed off. Then it stimulates the growth of new tissue. The treatment uses collagen taken from cattle, freeze-dried, and applied directly to a wound.

If you are at risk, talk to your doctor about this promising new treatment.

———————

Magnets may master foot pain

Suffering from peripheral neuropathy means constant tingling, burning pain, and even dangerous numbness in your feet. To help cope, you may have tried every remedy in the book. But here's a treatment that may be new to you.

For years, magnets have been promoted as a cure for everything from arthritis to impotence to hemorrhoids. Now, information from New York Medical College states that diabetics may get some relief from their disabling foot pain if they wear magnetic foot insoles 24 hours a day.

In this small four-month study, 90 percent of the diabetics had considerably less pain and burning while wearing the insoles. Their symptoms returned, however, when they stopped. Researchers believe more studies are needed before they can recommend this type of treatment, but they also believe magnetotherapy is generally safe.

Talk to your doctor before trying this alternative therapy. Certain health conditions, such as pregnancy or wearing a pacemaker, can have dangerous effects from magnets. In addition, the FDA does not endorse the use of magnets to treat medical problems. If you decide magnetic insoles are worth a try, you can find them at larger drug stores or on the Internet.

Caution: Inserts may be harmful to your feet

If you use any type of foot insoles, including magnetic ones, make sure they have a smooth surface, cautions Sean Ison, a board-certified pedorthist at a Dunwoody, Georgia shoe store. Ison designs and fits custom-made and prescriptive shoes and is concerned about inserts with a bumpy texture designed to stimulate or massage the feet.

"The problem with diabetic neuropathy," he says, "is that your feet have no sensation. After walking on the lumps and bumps on these insoles, a sore spot could develop that you wouldn't even notice. A sore spot can start an ulcer which can easily progress into something much worse."

Ison deals with many diabetics with foot problems and always designs their shoe surfaces to be soft and safe. If you stick with smooth surfaces that conform to your feet, he says inserts shouldn't cause you any problems.

On the road with diabetes —
20 tips for safe and easy travel

Going out of town on business? Planning a sightseeing excursion, a visit to relatives, or just some time to leave all your worries behind? Enjoy the trip, but remember — you won't be leaving your diabetes behind. Whether traveling by road, sea, air, or rail, you have special concerns you need to think about and plan for in order to have a smooth, enjoyable holiday.

Plan before you go. Take some time to get organized. If you're prepared, even the unexpected can't spoil your good time.

▶ Visit your doctor at least four to six weeks before your scheduled departure, and get a thorough exam. Discuss vaccinations, how to adjust your insulin or medication to different time zones, what travel medications you should have, and if there are specific food or drink concerns while in another country. Find out about special devices (pre-filled syringes, injection "pens," or pumps) that could make traveling easier.

▶ Get an official letter from your doctor documenting your condition. This will explain your needles and syringes to customs officials.

▶ Call the airline, rail line, or cruise ship in advance and order special meals. Check on this again the day of departure.

▶ Break in new shoes gradually and well in advance of your trip.

▶ Talk to a traveling companion about your condition and what she should do in case of an emergency.

▶ Review your health insurance policy to see if you are covered for medical care in other countries. If necessary, you can purchase separate coverage for foreign travel.

▶ If you are traveling to a non-English-speaking country, learn a few important phrases before you go, such as, "I need a doctor," "I have diabetes," and "I need sugar."

Pack smart. It can mean the difference between a trip that's frantic and one that's relaxed.

▶ Take enough insulin or medications to last your entire trip, plus some extra if possible. Insulin doesn't need to be refrigerated, but it should be protected from extreme heat and cold. Packing it inside a wide-mouthed thermos may be a good idea.

▶ Delays are just a part of traveling. Be prepared with snacks (canned juice, dried fruits, cheese, peanut butter, crackers, nuts, etc.) and emergency sugar cubes or packets in case of hypoglycemia.

▶ Divide your insulin, medications, and snacks between your checked luggage and your carry-on.

▶ Wear your diabetes ID tag or bracelet at all times.

▶ Make sure you've got insulin dose information, copies of prescriptions, insurance identification card, and your regular doctor's name and number in your wallet.

▶ Put together a small medicine kit. Be sure to include basic items like antiseptics and Band-Aids for blisters. Traveler's diarrhea can be a particular problem for you. Talk to your doctor about antibiotics you can take beforehand and include an over-the-counter anti-diarrheal medicine for emergencies.

Stay in control. While you're traveling, think about ways to stay comfortable and keep your diabetes under control.

▶ Dress in loose, comfortable clothes and shoes.

▶ Adjust your insulin as you go through time zones, according to your doctor's instructions.

▶ Move around as much as possible. Get up and stretch; take a stroll through the plane, bus, or train; if possible, stop, get out, and walk around.

▶ Consider keeping a travel diary. Include when and what you eat and a record of your blood glucose levels. In case you develop a problem, this may help identify the cause. It could also make your next trip easier to plan.

Relax when you get there. Don't get too caught up in the excitement of new places and new schedules.

▶ Don't forget to eat. Stick to a meal schedule, and plan ahead so you're not stranded somewhere without a restaurant in sight.

▶ Pay even more attention to your feet. They're probably getting a harder workout than usual. A little TLC now can prevent a lot of problems tomorrow.

▶ Stock up on the kind of blood glucose testing strips that you're familiar with, and check your blood sugar levels frequently. If your routine and physical activities are different, your body may respond differently as well.

For more information on travel and diabetes, contact the American Diabetes Association (800-232-3472) or the ADA Patient Information Hotline (800-342-2383). You can visit the association's website at www.diabetes.org.

Diverticulosis

How to dodge diverticulosis

Chances are, you're going to have diverticulosis someday. You may even have it now. Half the people over age 60 have the pea-sized pouches along the large intestine walls called diverticula.

But it's not a problem as long as they don't bother you. It's when the diverticula become infected and inflamed that you may begin to regret the diet habits that gave you those pouches. Infected diverticula can cause cramps, pain, tenderness in the left side of your stomach, gas, and blood in your stools. That's called diverticulitis. But you can keep the pouches from growing in the first place by changing your diet to include less fat and red meat and more fiber.

Sacrifice the steak. Researchers believe red meat causes bacteria in your intestines to weaken your colon and make it easier for diverticula to form. Fish and chicken don't seem to have this effect.

The fat in meat is also a problem. Researchers have found that fat from other sources, like dairy, is much less likely to lead to diverticulosis than fat from red meat. In fact, one study of 50,000 doctors showed that those who ate a lot of fatty meat and not much fiber were most likely to develop painful diverticulitis.

It may be tough to give up those juicy steaks, but doing so will help pave the way for problem-free digestion.

Learn to love grains. Fiber is the biggest key to fighting off diverticulosis because, quite simply, it makes things easy on your colon. Straining during bowel movements is a prime culprit in causing diverticula to form — by pushing out weak spots in the wall of your colon. Fiber softens your stool and keeps the pressure down in your bowels, so things move more smoothly. It also helps stimulate the muscles of your digestive tract, which keeps the walls of your intestines toned and healthy and less likely to giveout.

The American Dietetic Association says you should eat 20 to 35 grams of fiber every day. The World Health Organization recommends 27 to 40 grams. Grains are possibly the best sources for adding fiber to your diet. Try these fiber powerhouses, but keep in mind, the more a grain is processed, the less benefit you get.

▶ **Bran.** The outer husk of grains, or bran, is the greatest source of grain fiber you can eat. You can find bran in everything from cereals and breads to snack foods.

▶ **Barley.** This is also a good source of fiber, but keep an eye on what kind you buy. Whole-grain barley has 31 grams of fiber per cup, while pearl barley has only six. Why? Processing.

▶ **Oats.** You'll see this grain in many forms, but oat bran is probably your best bet for fiber-packing power. Just one-third of a cup provides 5 grams of fiber.

▶ **Other grains.** Experiment with other, less-common grain sources such as wild rice, rice bran, rice flour, rye flour, semolina, bulgur, millet, and buckwheat grass. They'll add some pizzazz to your everyday menu.

Enjoy your fruits and veggies. Grains aren't the only name in the high-fiber game. Fruits and vegetables encourage the growth of microbes in your intestines that aid digestion. These microbes keep things "moving along," making it harder for diverticula to form or become infected. Some of your best bets in the fruit category are blackberries (6.6 grams per cup), raspberries (5.8), blueberries (4.4), dates, pears, and apples.

On the vegetable side, beans and peas are your strongest ally. Broad beans are the best (8.7 grams per cup), followed by lentils, black beans, limas, pintos, baked, kidneys, all the way down to green peas, chickpeas, and black-eyed peas (4.4 grams).

One thing to remember about fiber — when you add more to your diet, be sure to take it slow. Sudden increases can make you feel bloated and gassy. Also, fiber absorbs a lot of water, and you must replace it or risk dehydration. Guard against this by drinking one-and-a-half to two quarts of water every day.

Keep your diet healthy by filling up on fiber and cutting back on red meat, and your intestines will reward you by staying smooth and inflammation free.

Popping the popcorn myth

For many years, doctors have warned their patients with diverticulosis against eating foods that have small seeds or tiny parts that could be hard to digest. Maybe you have felt your own spirits sink when informed that these "blacklisted" foods include such favorites as popcorn, tomatoes, and strawberries.

The reasoning was that such small particles could easily get caught in the diverticula on their way through the colon and cause the swelling or infection that leads to diverticulitis.

Even though some doctors still insist this advice is for the best, most now feel these danger foods are not a problem. In fact, according to the National Institute of Diabetes and Digestive and Kidney Diseases, there is no documented evidence to back up the popcorn myth.

Don't be tempted by the quick fix

Think laxatives or painkillers are the answer to the discomfort of diverticulosis? Think again. Although you might see laxatives as a quick way to eliminate constipation — one of the main causes of those irritating intestinal sacs — they can lead to many other problems. And painkillers like aspirin and ibuprofen may actually make your diverticulosis worse.

Leave laxatives alone. Many over-the-counter laxatives are designed to make your bowels contract, which can further irritate your colon. Laxatives also interfere with your body's ability to absorb the nutrients it needs from foods, and some researchers believe they can even weaken your resistance to heart disease and cancer. Worse still, laxatives can become addictive.

The best solution is to let nature take its course with help from a high-fiber, low-fat diet, complete with plenty of water. If you feel you need a little extra push once in a while, try a natural softener like prunes, prune juice, or psyllium. But avoid products with senna, which is a strong herbal laxative.

Say no to NSAIDs. You may pop an aspirin or Advil when intestinal pain flares, but that may not be the best thing to do. At least one study has shown that non-steroidal anti-inflammatory drugs (NSAIDs) like these may lead to severe complications in people with diverticulosis.

The study at the University of Aberdeen compared the severity of diverticular disease among three groups: people with severe complications, people with no complications, and people without diverticular disease. Almost 50 percent of those with severe complications were taking NSAIDs, compared with an average of 19 percent among the other groups.

Researchers believe this difference is enough to show that taking NSAIDs regularly may result in a more serious form of diverticular disease. If you fall into this category — particularly if you are over 60 or know you have diverticulosis — talk to your doctor about what you can do to lower your risk.

Drug Reactions

7 ways to sidestep deadly drug errors

Camilla Yates, a pregnant woman with gestational diabetes, picked up her first prescription for insulin at her usual drug store. Since she had just read an article on the importance of checking prescriptions, she compared the label to what the doctor had written.

"I was shocked," she said. "My pharmacist misread 5U as 50 and wrote my insulin instructions as 'take 50 units' instead of five units. I can't imagine what would have happened if I'd taken my first dose at 10 times the amount called for."

Luckily, Camilla noticed the error in time to avert a deadly disaster for her and her baby. Many people aren't so fortunate. According to a study published in the Journal of the American Medical Association, more than 100,000 people die every year from adverse drug reactions. That makes it between the fourth and sixth leading cause of death in the United States.

Don't be frightened into throwing away all your prescriptions, however. Medications also save many lives every year, and you can take steps to avoid becoming a victim to your prescription.

Write down the prescription. Copy the generic and brand names of your prescription, plus dosing information, while you're at your doctor's office. Then you'll have a record, in your own handwriting, to check against your actual prescription when you get it filled. Many times prescription errors occur because the pharmacist can't read the doctor's handwriting.

Inform your doctor. Make sure you tell your doctor about any other medications you're taking. Don't assume he knows, even if he prescribed your other medicines. Include any over-the-counter medications, herbs, or supplements. And remind him of any drug allergies you have. Often, people who are allergic to one drug may also be allergic to a related drug.

Stick with the same pharmacy. Most pharmacies now have computerized systems that will warn you if you've been prescribed two drugs that may interact. If you go to different pharmacies, however, you lose that advantage.

Check your pills. When you get a refill, check to make sure the pills look like the ones you're used to taking. If there is a change, ask your pharmacist about it.

Schedule a "brown bag" session. Put every medicine you're taking into a bag and let your doctor or pharmacist examine them for potential interactions, duplication, or expired dates.

Skip the alcohol. Alcohol is a drug that can interact with many prescription medications. To be safe, if you're taking medication, stay away from alcohol.

Don't be afraid to ask questions. Make sure you understand what you're taking and why. Your doctor and pharmacist want you to stay healthy, so they'll be glad to answer any questions you have.

Life-saving advice for the elderly

Even properly prescribed medicine can be dangerous if you don't take it properly. That can be a particular problem for the elderly.

Older adults are more likely to take several types of medication, increasing the risk of interactions. And because their reading vision often declines as they age, they're more likely to misread the fine print on prescription labels. If vision is a problem for you, don't be embarrassed to ask your pharmacist to give your instructions in large print.

You also may have problems remembering whether or not you've taken your medication. This uncertainty might result in your taking too little or too much medicine, perhaps even causing an overdose. Containers that divide your dosages up for the week can be helpful.

Focusing on your pill while you take it is another good way to help yourself remember, according to psychologist Gilles

Einstein. Don't just swallow it quickly; swish it around in your mouth, and make a mental note of it. You'll be more likely to remember you took it and maybe save yourself from a dangerous overdose.

Harness the power of the placebo

In his classic book *The Power of Positive Thinking*, Norman Vincent Peale emphasizes how your mind and attitude can affect your life, including your health.

A good example is the placebo effect. A placebo is a harmless, unmedicated pill often given to a patient to "humor" him. The amazing thing is some people, unaware they are taking a placebo, actually start feeling better. Many doctors think these people get better because they expect to get better.

Studies show up to 70 percent of people with depression who receive a placebo improve, but those who get no treatment rarely do. Just the act of taking the "medicine" can help, whether or not it contains anything beneficial.

In another study, people with asthma were given an inhaler that only contained harmless salt water. When they were told the inhaler contained an allergen, their airway obstruction increased, and they had more difficulty breathing. When told the same inhaler contained medication, their airways opened up, and they could breathe more easily.

Even the color of the pill can have an effect. Research shows that people expect blue or green pills to have a calming effect and red, yellow, or orange pills to have a stimulating effect. In one study, people were told they were taking either a sedative or a stimulant, but they were actually given pink or blue placebos. Twice as many people taking the blue pills reported drowsiness as those who took the pink pills.

The placebo effect has great healing potential. To harness this power, find a competent doctor and have confidence in his ability to help you. This will boost your chances of getting better. The power of the placebo may be the same as the power of positive thinking.

Herbs and drugs can be a deadly duo

Most people use alternative medicine in addition to conventional medicine. This blending of the modern and the ancient can be very beneficial, but it can also be dangerous. Some drugs and herbs that are safe when taken alone can cause dangerous side effects when taken together.

If you're taking a supplement, ask your doctor if it could interact with a prescription drug you are taking. Here are a few potential problems to watch out for.

▶ **Ginkgo.** Many herbalists recommend ginkgo to improve your memory. Ginkgo works by improving blood flow to your brain. It widens your blood vessels and makes your platelets less sticky. If you are taking a daily aspirin or an anticoagulant, like warfarin or heparin, don't use ginkgo. It could magnify the blood-thinning effect. Epileptics who take anticonvulsants, like carbamazepine, phenytoin, and phenobarbital, shouldn't take ginkgo because it might reduce the effectiveness of those medications.

▶ **Echinacea.** One of the best-selling herbs, echinacea is thought to boost your immune system, making it especially popular during cold and flu season. If you have an autoimmune disorder, like lupus or rheumatoid arthritis, you shouldn't take echinacea. It can counteract the effects of your medication. Echinacea, if taken for long periods of time, loses its effectiveness and may cause liver damage. For that reason, don't take echinacea with any medication that has liver damage as a potential side effect.

▶ **Ginger**. This well-known stomach soother helps prevent nausea caused by motion sickness. A study at the University of Alabama revealed that it even helps ease the nausea caused by chemotherapy. Because it also has blood-thinning qualities, don't take it if you're taking an anticoagulant.

▶ **Ginseng.** In Eastern medicine, ginseng is known as an "adaptogen." This means it strengthens your body's resistance to unhealthy influences and works to keep it in balance. Studies have found that it has a favorable effect on the blood sugar levels of diabetics. Ginseng shouldn't be used with anticoagulants, like warfarin and heparin, or nonsteroidal anti-inflammatory drugs (NSAIDs), like ibuprofen and aspirin. It may also cause problems if taken with corticosteroids.

▶ **St. John's wort.** Studies show this herbal supplement is an effective treatment for mild to moderate depression. Its one notable side effect is increased sensitivity to the sun. In addition to limiting your sunbathing, don't combine it with other medication that could make your skin more sensitive to the sun. St. John's wort shouldn't be taken with prescription antidepressants, particularly MAO inhibitors.

▶ **Feverfew.** This herb has been used to treat migraine headaches for almost 2,000 years. Modern studies show it's effective in reducing the number and severity of migraine attacks. Nonsteroidal anti-inflammatory drugs (NSAIDs), like ibuprofen and aspirin, can reduce feverfew's effectiveness. Don't take feverfew if you're allergic to ragweed, yarrow, or chamomile. Those plants are in the same family, and you'd probably be allergic to feverfew, too.

▶ **Valerian.** This herb can help you get a good night's sleep, but don't take it if you're drinking alcohol. Experts aren't sure if valerian interacts with alcohol. To be on the safe side, don't combine the two. Since valerian prolongs the effects of barbiturates, like thiopental and pentobarbital, it shouldn't be taken with any barbiturate.

More dangerous drug-herb interactions

Herb	Drugs that may cause interactions
Bromelain	Anticoagulants (warfarin, heparin) and NSAIDs (aspirin, ibuprofen)
Garlic	Anticoagulants (warfarin, heparin) and NSAIDs (aspirin, ibuprofen)
Licorice	Digoxin, MAO inhibitors, may counteract cyclosporine
Hawthorn	Digoxin
Kava kava	Alprazolam
Evening primrose oil	Anticonvulsants
Chamomile	Anticoagulants (warfarin, heparin) and NSAIDs (aspirin, ibuprofen)
Saw palmetto	Hormonal therapies (estrogen replacement therapy, birth control pills)
Ephedra	Stimulants

A consumer's guide to buying supplements

When Mary Watkins started having pain in her knees, her doctor told her she had osteoarthritis. He prescribed painkillers, but Mary was concerned about taking them every day. "My niece recommended some supplement that was supposed to be good for arthritis, but I couldn't remember the name of it," she said. "I went to the drugstore and was just overwhelmed. I had no idea there were so many different supplements for sale."

The number of products available wasn't the only reason for Mary's confusion. "I spent about 20 minutes standing in front of this huge display, but I couldn't find any products that said they could help arthritis."

That's because the DSHEA (Dietary Supplement Health and Education Act) allows the unrestricted sale of vitamins, minerals, herbs, amino acids, and other dietary supplements, as long as the manufacturers don't make medical claims for their products.

Although this protects you from unproven and false medical claims, it can make buying supplements confusing.

For example, glucosamine sulfate, the product Mary's niece recommended, is a supplement that studies show helps rebuild cartilage in your joints, which relieves arthritis symptoms. However, manufacturers of glucosamine sulfate can't say it "improves arthritis." They can only make claims about how their product affects certain body structures and functions. For instance, a glucosamine sulfate label might say, "promotes joint health."

The best way to know what to buy is to do your homework. You can learn a lot by talking with a reputable herbalist. Don't depend on salesclerks to help you pick out products. Some of them are knowledgeable, but many don't know anything about the supplements they're selling.

Here are a few items to consider when shopping for supplements.

▶ Look for standardized products. Whole herb products can vary greatly in their potency, depending on where they were grown, soil and weather conditions, and other variables. Standardized products have a set percentage of the active ingredient in a particular herb. For example, kava products, which are used to relieve stress, are standardized to contain 30 percent kavalactones.

▶ Make sure you read labels carefully and take any manufacturer's warnings into account. Just because it's natural doesn't mean it's safe for everyone. Many products carry cautions for pregnant or nursing women, and some products aren't recommended for people with certain conditions, like diabetes or high blood pressure.

▶ Pay attention to your body's reaction to any supplement you take. It's a good idea to try one new product at a time. If you have an adverse reaction, you'll have a better idea what might have caused it.

▶ Tell your doctor what supplements you're taking. Some supplements can interact with prescription drugs.

Dry Eyes

10 soothing remedies for dry eyes

The eyes, some say, are the windows to the soul. But when your "windows" feel gritty and scratchy, it can really dull your spirit. Normally, your body bathes your eyes in soothing teardrops. But if you have the condition called dry eyes, you may feel like they are being rubbed with sandpaper instead.

Itchy, red, swollen eyes are probably the symptoms you notice first. You also may be bothered by blurred vision and a burning sensation. A stringy mucus might form in your eyes, and wearing contact lenses can become unbearable.

Tears may not come even when you feel like crying. But, on the other hand, you may find your eyes are watery. This seems a strange symptom of dry eyes, but healthy tears contain oil and mucus. Water alone doesn't coat and cling to your eyes properly. Instead, it evaporates quickly, leaving them unprotected and dry.

You are more likely to experience dry eyes if you are:

▶ over 40 — especially if you are a woman who has passed menopause

▶ have allergies

▶ wear contact lenses

▶ spend a lot of time at the computer

▶ do close reading or other detail work

Your dry eyes also could be caused by Sjogren's syndrome, especially if you experience dry mouth as well. This is a serious autoimmune disorder that destroys the glands that produce tears and saliva. In addition to the other symptoms of dry eyes, people with Sjogren's often notice that fluorescent light really bothers them. An eye doctor can test your eyes to determine if this is the cause of your problem.

Fortunately, most of the time dry eyes is a temporary condition. Usually all you need to do is give your eyes a good rest, and they'll be moist and comfortable again. Following these soothing remedies should help put the twinkle back in your eyes.

Avoid irritants from the environment. Try to stay away from smoke, toxic fumes, and other pollutants that can bother your eyes. You may even need to leave off your eye make-up, or at least reduce the amount you use.

Add some moisture. Dry air means dry eyes. So add moisture to the air in your home or office with a humidifier. You'll also find it helpful to drink extra water, especially when flying. Airplane cabins tend to have extra-dry air.

Don't rub it in. It's such a temptation to dig at those itchy eyes, but dry eyes are easily infected. "Hands off" is the best policy.

Protect your peepers. Dry eyes are sensitive to bright light, so wear sunglasses when you go outside. You may even want to wear swim or ski goggles or moisture chamber glasses, especially if Sjogren's syndrome is the cause of your problem. They help to prevent moisture from evaporating as quickly.

Take a break and blink. Do you spend a lot of time reading, using a computer, or doing other close work? You are less likely to blink when performing these tasks, and if you don't, your eyes will suffer. So bat those eyelashes as often as possible.

Use artificial tears. For occasional, short-term use, try tear substitutes. They soothe and protect your eyes just like real tears do. But don't use them too often or they'll interrupt your eyes' natural tear production. You should also avoid products that contain preservatives, which can make the problem worse.

Instead of liquid drops, you might prefer to use an ointment. Because it's thicker and stickier, it will stay on the surface of your eye longer. Use ointments at bedtime because they can blur your vision. You can also get long-lasting soluble inserts. Lacrisert is an example of one without preservatives. You place this tiny pellet inside your lower eyelid where it melts slowly over six to eight hours and helps thicken your tears.

Be careful with contacts. If you wear contact lenses, be especially careful about what you put in your eyes. Drops and ointments may make your eyes more comfortable, but they could mask a serious problem with the contacts themselves.

As a rule, stick with a rewetting solution designed for use with your brand of contacts, or use medications recommended by your eye doctor. In most cases, you'll need to remove the contacts before applying any medication. Follow the doctor's instructions or the package directions about how long to wait before replacing them.

Get plenty of vitamin A. This vitamin is essential for healthy eyes. You'll find it in meat and dairy products. Also, plant sources like leafy green vegetables are high in beta carotene, which converts to vitamin A in your body. You can get vitamin A through supplements, but too much can be dangerous. A daily multiple vitamin will safely provide what you need.

Monitor your medications. Your dry eyes could be caused by medicines you take. Decongestants, diuretics, general anesthetics, beta-adrenergic blockers, antimuscarinics, and thiabendazole are likely culprits. Talk to your regular doctor about your situation. Perhaps another medication would do just as well without this side effect.

See your doctor often. Regular checkups are important to your eyes' health. And if dry eyes don't clear up quickly or are a chronic problem, you'll need to see your eye doctor more often. You could have damage to the eye or a blocked tear duct that needs treatment by an ophthalmologist.

Simple eye drop solution

Do you find that liquid eye drops just run down your cheeks like tears? Do you dodge the dropper or squint your eye closed just before the drop hits? Or if using eye ointment, do you get more smeared around your eyes than in them?

If these misses sound familiar, these guidelines can help you avoid the messes. A hint: Make sure you put the drops inside your bottom eyelid — don't try to splash them against your eyeball. And, of course, always begin with clean hands.

► Tilt your head back slightly with eyes open. Looking up toward the ceiling will reduce the urge to blink. It also lowers the chance that the drops will sting. You can also delay any irritation slightly by using cold eye drops.

► Make a pocket with your lower eyelid by placing your middle or index finger just under your bottom lashes and pulling down gently.

► Apply a single drop of liquid or a small amount of ointment into the pocket. Be careful not to touch your eye with the applicator. You may want to place the hand holding the dropper firmly against your face or other hand to keep it steady.

► Give the drops or ointment a few moments to settle inside the lid. Then slowly close your eyes and gently roll them around to coat the entire lens. Don't squeeze them tight or you might force out some of the solution.

► Open your eyes slowly, and blink once to mix the solution with your natural tears. Then close your eye for 30 seconds to allow the solution to stick to the surface of your eyeball.

► Wipe excess liquid or ointment from eyelashes and eyelids with a soft cloth or tissue.

You may prefer to insert the drops or ointment while lying down if tilting your head back makes you dizzy. This will also be helpful if you've recently had eye surgery.

Certain medications or health conditions may require different instructions. For example, you may need to prevent the drops from draining into your tear duct, nose, or throat. You can do this by pressing your index finger against the inside corner of your eye (beside your nose) for a minute or two after the drops go in.

Always ask your doctor or pharmacist if there are any special instructions with your eye medications, and be sure to follow them carefully.

Drop anti-redness eye drops

You look into the mirror and see bloodshot eyes staring back at you. Not a pretty sight! Your first thought is to run out and buy some non-prescription eye drops that promise to "get the red out."

But wait. These solutions may make matters worse. Researchers looked at 70 people who developed pink eye (conjunctivitis) after using eye drops. It turned out their inflammation was caused by the naphazoline, tetrahydrozoline, or phenylephrine in the eye drops. These drugs are vasoconstrictors that cause your blood vessels to shrink, allowing less oxygen to get to your eyes.

When people stopped using the drops, their eyes cleared up, in most cases, after a few weeks. But sometimes there is a rebound effect, and the condition gets worse before it gets better.

So play it smart when it comes to eye drops. Don't use them for long periods, and stop if your eyes feel worse. Also, consider other remedies. You may be better off using tear substitutes that soothe your red eyes but don't have ingredients that make them worse.

Dry Mouth

6 tips for dealing with dry mouth

Everyone has felt that awful apprehension before a special event that causes your stomach to flutter and your mouth to go dry — nothing is more of a nuisance.

Many prescription or over-the-counter medications also make your mouth feel as dry as the Sahara. Drugs for depression, high blood pressure, pain, weight loss, and flu or cold symptoms especially leave you parched.

Dehydration, heat exhaustion, salty foods, infected salivary glands, diabetes, or simply getting older — these are all common causes of dry mouth. But if you're a post-menopausal woman over 50 who suddenly finds her mouth and eyes dry, you may be suffering from a condition called Sjogren's (show-grins) syndrome.

This is a disease in which your immune system attacks your moisture-producing glands so you don't create as much saliva or tears as you need. It's not a life-threatening condition, but it does get progressively worse, and it can damage your eyes and mouth if the symptoms aren't treated.

Saliva is important to your health because it cleans your mouth of bacteria, helps heal wounds or sores, and keeps your mouth lubricated. Without it, you'll have problems talking and eating, and you may develop painful mouth sores, fungal infections, and tooth decay.

There is no known cure for Sjogren's syndrome, but you can head off problems and ease your symptoms with a little planning and know-how.

> ▶ **Practice good oral hygiene.** Brush your teeth, or at least rinse out your mouth, every time you eat. Use a soft toothbrush, perhaps even an electric one. Try a device that uses

water to irrigate your mouth. Floss regularly but gently. Use home fluoride treatments and fluoride toothpaste. See your dentist more often — maybe three or four times a year — for a checkup, thorough cleaning, and fluoride treatment.

► **Avoid alcohol, caffeine and smoking.** They dry out your membranes.

► **Get your juices flowing.** Chew sugarless gum (especially those containing the sugar substitute xylitol), drink sugar-free sodas, or suck on hard candy or lemons.

► **Drink plenty of liquids.** Sip throughout the day but especially with meals. This will help moisten your food, making it easier for you to swallow. Milk is a good choice since it seems to coat and soothe your mouth and can help prevent tooth decay.

► **Control your air quality.** Use a humidifier to moisten the air, and avoid air conditioning and heated air whenever possible — they are both drying.

► **Send in a substitute.** You can also take advantage of several products designed to substitute for your own saliva. They are the most effective way to moisten a severely parched throat and mouth. Some even contain fluoride to protect your teeth from decay. Look for those with the American Dental Association seal of approval.

Whether your dry mouth is a result of chronic illness or just a temporary challenge, it's an aggravating aspect of life. But today, more than ever before, you have a variety of ways to make your dry mouth feel normal again.

Dry Skin

Dry skin remedies by the dozen

You know that scaly, itchy, dry sensation that means your skin will soon be molting like a garden snake. You can feel it from your lips to your feet and everywhere in between. Although it happens most often in winter, when indoor air is heated and dry and you tend to use hotter water, it can happen any time. Whether your irritated skin is from sunburn and swimming, spring cleaning and detergents, or just plain aging, try these tips for relief.

Be cool. Wash your skin with warm or cool water — never hot.

Soak up some softness. Baths are actually less drying to your skin than showers — as long as you use warm water and don't soak longer than 10 minutes.

Take a break. Try to bathe every other day or even just a few times a week. This will reduce how often you strip the protective oils from your skin.

Heat the air, not the water. Warm up your bathroom — with a space heater if necessary — so you'll feel more comfortable bathing in cooler water.

Choose a mild soap. Save the strong, antibacterial deodorant soaps for your underarms, feet, and genital area.

Stop scrubbing. Don't rub your skin too hard after bathing. In fact, patting or blotting with a soft towel is best.

Moisturize. Pat on a lotion right after your bath or shower to lock in moisture.

Avoid the elements. Don't expose your skin to too much sun, wind, or cold.

Go tropical. Avoid dry air if possible. Keep a humidifier running in your home or office.

Balance your diet. Eat plenty of foods containing vitamins A and C to keep your skin smooth and supple. For vitamin A, choose dark green and orange fruits and vegetables, meat, and dairy products. To get extra vitamin C, eat citrus fruits, peppers, strawberries, and other fruits and vegetables.

Turn on the tap. Drink lots of water every day — at least three large glasses.

Don't forget your fingers. Wear gloves when you do housework or dishes to protect your hands from drying chemicals and hot water.

If you're still not able to beat the dryness or annoying itch, visit a dermatologist. He can prescribe special creams, ointments, or even an oral antihistamine. He'll also try to find out what's causing your problem — allergies, a drug reaction, or some other condition.

Dermatologists' #1 choice for treating dry skin

Petrolatum, a thick, jelly-like substance made from petroleum, is considered by many dermatologists to be the most effective moisturizer. It has been proven to reduce the amount of water lost from your skin by about 50 percent. In addition, it protects your skin from irritants and is more deeply absorbed than other moisturizers.

Dr. James T. Sandwich of Fayette Area Dermatology in Georgia says that, when used appropriately, it's a wonderful emollient. "It does a good job of keeping moisture in the skin. If you have dry skin or a condition, like eczema, caused by not enough oil in your skin, petrolatum traps moisture to hydrate your skin."

"It's a little bit greasy," he adds, "so sometimes it's not as elegant as some of the other moisturizers. But still it's a good product."

Sandwich warns that petrolatum should not be used over wounds that are weeping or infected. It creates too much of a barrier and does not allow toxins to escape. "But with very dry skin," he says, "you've got cracks that allow foreign material and bacteria to come in contact with the skin in deeper areas than normal.

The petrolatum, as long as it's put on in a thin film, doesn't allow things to get into those cracks."

Some moisturizers that contain petrolatum are:

- Oil of Olay Daily Renewal Moisturizing Body Wash
- Jergens Ultra Healing Lotion
- Pacquin Plus with Aloe Skin Cream
- Desitin Ointment
- Lubriderm Seriously Sensitive Lotion

Soothe skin problems with healing herbs

Herbs have been used since the beginning of time for healing, comfort, flavor, and every cosmetic purpose from war paint to make-up. Whether your goal is timeless beauty or timely first aid, an herbal remedy may be just what your dry or irritated skin needs.

Aloe vera. Aloe is perhaps the most well-known plant for healing skin irritations and wounds. You'll find it growing in small flower pots in kitchens around the country since the gel taken from a freshly cut leaf is a super remedy for minor burns. Aloe is also a major ingredient in dozens of commercial skin products, from moisturizing lotions to after-sun soothers.

Calendula. This herb, also known as common marigold, has yellow or orange flowers that are a familiar sight in many gardens and flower beds. Not only will calendula brighten your home, you can use it to treat mild skin irritations.

A cream or ointment is commonly made from the calendula flower heads and rubbed on your skin to heal rashes, inflammations, or minor wounds.

Capsaicin. If you suffer from psoriasis, you'll want to try capsaicin cream. Made from the potent ingredient in cayenne pepper, it may surprise you at first with its fiery sensation on your skin. Most people find the long-term benefits are worth any initial discomfort.

Chamomile. A member of the daisy family, chamomile is perhaps most widely used as a soothing herbal tea. But in Germany, chamomile cream was found to be almost as effective as hydrocortisone at healing dermatitis, skin ulcers, and other minor irritations.

Witch hazel. If your skin is itchy or inflamed, reach for a bottle of witch hazel. It has been used for years to soothe various skin problems, including dermatitis.

Unfortunately, the distilled witch hazel most commonly available in the United States contains such a small amount of volatile oil that it has almost no healing properties. When buying witch hazel, look for authentic or nondistilled hydroalcoholic extract of witch hazel leaves. It should contain from 5 to 10 percent leaf extract.

Enlarged Prostate

Walking lowers your risk of BPH

Dave Robbins couldn't sleep through the night. "I felt like a baby," he said. "I had to get up two or three times a night to go to the bathroom. At first I thought I was getting diabetes, because it runs in my family, but then I went to the doctor and found out I had BPH."

Many men like Dave discover that a tiny body part called the prostate can cause big problems, especially as men get older. Half of men over age 60 — and 90 percent of men over age 85 — develop an enlarged prostate or benign prostatic hyperplasia (BPH).

BPH causes urinary problems because of the prostate's location — right around the urethra, the tube that carries urine from your bladder out of your body. When your prostate becomes enlarged, it puts the squeeze on your urethra, making it more difficult to urinate.

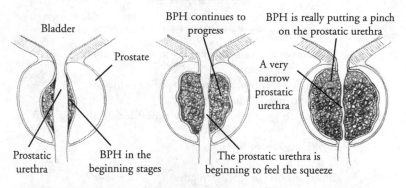

Although BPH is usually more of a nuisance than a danger, it can lead to more serious problems. When urine can't get through your urethra, it has no place to go but back up into your bladder. There it often stagnates and causes urinary tract and bladder infections. You may also develop painful bladder stones or experience sexual difficulties. Untreated BPH can even lead to kidney damage because of increased pressure on the kidneys or the spread of infection from the bladder to the kidneys.

If you want to reduce your risk of developing BPH, a brisk walk a few times around the block could help. A recent study found that active men were 25 percent less likely to have moderate to severe symptoms of the disorder or to have had surgery for BPH than less active men. Walking just two to three hours a week was enough exercise to bring about this level of risk reduction, but adding another three hours of walking per week reduced risk by another 10 percent.

Another reason to exercise is to keep off excess weight. According to a five-year study of more than 25,000 men, being 35 pounds or more overweight or gaining more than seven inches in your waist increases your risk of BPH by 75 percent after age 50. In fact, by age 75 to 80, about half the men with a waist size larger than 43 inches had moderate to severe urinary problems, with some of them even requiring surgery. On the other hand, only about one-third of the men with a waist size of 35 inches or less had significant urinary difficulties.

Symptoms of BPH

- Difficulty getting urine stream to start; hesitancy
- Weak urine stream
- Feeling of incomplete emptying after urination
- Frequent need to urinate
- Having to get up one or more times during the night to urinate
- Dribbling, incontinence
- Insomnia
- Interruptions in urine stream

No-surgery solutions to prostate enlargement

In Europe, at least 30 compounds containing active ingredients from plants are used to treat benign prostatic hyperplasia (BPH). In 70 percent of studies, plants have been found to be more effective than a placebo. In fact, some studies suggest plant remedies may help up to 80 percent of the men using them. The major advantage of plant remedies over manufactured drugs is the much lower risk of serious side effects.

Here are some of the more common remedies used to treat BPH. If you choose to use any of these remedies, let your doctor know. He still needs to monitor your prostate.

Saw palmetto. Berries from a small palm tree that grows in the southeastern United States could help relieve your BPH. Several studies have found that a concentrated extract of saw palmetto berries can relieve the symptoms of BPH. A recent review of these studies found that compared with a placebo, saw palmetto improved overall urinary symptoms by 28 percent. Two of the studies reviewed found that saw palmetto was as effective as finasteride, the main drug used to treat BPH, and caused fewer side effects.

If you would like to try saw palmetto, choose a supplement of lipophilic (fat-soluble) extract that contains 85 to 95 percent fatty acids. Experts recommend taking 160 milligrams (mg) twice daily or 320 mg once a day. It may take four to six weeks before you notice any improvement.

Stinging nettle. Another plant remedy that may ease the symptoms of BPH comes from the root and leaves of the stinging nettle. Many products combine stinging nettle and saw palmetto. One study on this combination found that 160 mg of saw palmetto and 120 mg of stinging nettle root extract taken twice daily improved urinary flow by 26 percent, reduced residual urine (urine left in your bladder after you urinate) by 45 percent, reduced pain during urination by 63 percent, reduced dribbling after urination by 54 percent, and cut nighttime trips to the bathroom by half.

Pumpkin seeds. A new and unusual remedy for prostate problems is pumpkin seeds. A handful of pumpkin seeds a day has long been used as a treatment for enlarged prostate in Bulgaria, Turkey, and the Ukraine. Now these seeds are popping up at health food stores everywhere. Although studies to support pumpkin seeds' claim to prostate fame are slim, pumpkin seeds are rich in zinc, an important mineral for prostate health.

Soy. Adding some soy foods, like tofu and soy milk, to your diet might be a healthy choice for your prostate. Research shows that isoflavones (hormone-like substances in soy) seem to stop, or at least slow down, the process of prostate enlargement. And if you cut the fat in your diet by adding some soy instead of fatty meats, you may also decrease your risk of BPH. Dietary fat can increase hormone production, which may stimulate prostate growth. Researchers speculate that eating a low-fat diet can protect you from these extra hormones.

Unfortunately, the soy picture is not all rosy. Many experts are concerned about the connection between soy and forgetfulness discovered several years ago. The research suggests soy makes your brain age faster — the more soy you eat, the greater your memory and learning difficulties, and the greater your risk of developing senility. While you don't have to avoid soy altogether, talk to your doctor about keeping to moderate amounts.

Eyestrain

RX for computer eyestrain

If your computer terminal has become a site for sore eyes, maybe it's time to invest in a pair of computer glasses. That's what researcher Kathleen Largo did, and it's made a world of difference in her job.

Although the computer is essential to her work in a Georgia publishing firm, Largo found it difficult to read the screen and was getting headaches as a result. She turned to her eye doctor, who fitted her with a pair of computer glasses. "They were exactly what I needed. I haven't had a headache since," she says.

Dr. Richard Lee, an ophthalmologist in Oakland, California, says problems often develop as you near age 40. That's when your lenses tend to lose a lot of flexibility and are unable to change shape the way they did when you were younger.

At this stage you may need bifocals, which usually work well for reading. But the part of the lens for close work is often too low for comfort at the computer terminal. If you are far-sighted, like Largo, this can be particularly frustrating.

"It's not as much trouble for near-sighted people," says Lee. "But people who are far-sighted need the screen to be a foot farther away."

Largo tried bifocals for a few months but found she was constantly moving her head trying to find the right spot for close viewing. "I couldn't get used to them," she says. "And I didn't want to give up headaches for neck problems."

According to Lee, the advantage of computer glasses is that the lenses are divided into two large halves, with the top half serving the purpose of the mid-range of trifocals. You use it for looking straight out at the screen, which is usually about two feet in front of you.

This area of the lens is much larger than what you have in trifocals, so the whole screen stays in view. And since you don't need distance vision at the computer, you have the entire bottom half for near-vision. You can look down at the full keyboard without twisting your head from side to side.

Studies show that computer-related vision problems are growing. Along with special glasses, the following tips can help your eyes stay alert and healthy:

► Position your computer and adjust your light to reduce glare.

► Use controls on your computer to adjust brightness and contrast to a level that's comfortable.

► Place work materials at the same distance as the screen.

► Stop about every 15 minutes and gaze off into the distance.

► Remember to blink frequently to keep your eyes moist.

Lee says that eyestrain won't weaken your eyesight or make eye diseases like cataracts or macular degeneration worse. But you can be more comfortable — and productive too — when you put an end to the worry of computer eyestrain.

Falling

7 ways to prevent falling

Each year, about one out of three people over the age of 65 falls. The injuries and complications from these falls often result in severe lifestyle changes. Many people are forced into nursing homes after a fall because they can no longer get around and care for themselves. Don't lose your independence because of a preventable accident. Take steps to protect yourself now.

Beware of the stairs. Make sure your staircases have handrails on both sides of the stairs, if possible, and use them. Cover your stairs with tight-knit carpeting or nonslip treads. And don't place things on lower steps that you plan to take upstairs later. Keep your stairs completely clutter-free.

Follow the path of least resistance. Arrange your furnishings so there is plenty of room to move around without having to go around or over obstacles. Keep throw rugs off the beaten path, and tuck all electrical cords safely out of harm's way.

Keep your floors and hallways clean. Wipe up any spills or tracked-in moisture immediately. Don't wax your kitchen floor or the hardwood in the hall. Waxed floors are slippery and dangerous. Keep muddy shoes, umbrellas, and other items out of high-traffic areas. They're just waiting to be tripped over.

Let there be light. Be sure your home is well lit, inside and out, particularly in areas of uneven or awkward footing, such as stairs. For security at night, keep a night-light burning in the bathroom, the bedroom, and wherever else you may roam.

Brace yourself in bed and bath. In the bathroom, use nonslip backing on bathmats and rugs. If your tub is slippery, put down nonslip tape to help you keep your footing. If you have trouble getting up and down, install a handrail in the tub and next to the toilet.

Don't lock your bedroom or bathroom door. If you fall and need help, you want help to be able to get to you.

Keep it down. Don't store things in high places that you need frequently. Whether it's your measuring cups in the kitchen or your favorite books in the family room, keep important items within easy reach. If you have to get something on a high shelf, always use a step stool, never a chair. If possible, get a step stool with handles.

Dress for success. Sensible shoes are a must for good balance. Avoid shoes that are unstable, like high heels and shoes with thick soles. Instead, go for snug, comfortable shoes with rubber soles and laces, and always keep your laces tied.

Being able to see also helps you avoid tripping over things. If you need glasses, wear them.

Take your time. Sitting up too fast upon waking, or jumping to your feet before you've had a chance to adjust to the light, can cause head rushes and dizziness. After sitting up in bed, wait for a few seconds on the side of the bed and get your bearings before standing.

To make this easier, and to avoid injury if you fall off the bed, use a bed that's not too far off the ground. If you can sit on the edge comfortably with your feet on the floor, that's a pretty convenient and safe height for you.

If, after all these precautions, you fall anyway, try to stay calm. Once you've composed yourself, check to see if you're hurt, and if so, how badly. If you can move comfortably, slide yourself to the nearest support — a chair or a wall — and try to stand. If you can't get yourself to your feet, crawl carefully to the phone and call friends or 911 for help.

Save your hips by knowing your risks

One of the best ways to lessen your risk of falling is to become familiar with the possible side effects of any medication you're taking.

Ask your doctor or pharmacist if the drugs you are taking could cause drowsiness or dizziness.

Antidepressants, in particular, have been associated with a greater risk of falling, especially among senior citizens. If you're taking an antidepressant, you've probably heard the recent outcry against SSRIs (selective serotonin reuptake inhibitors). Some studies claim that this type of antidepressant creates a greater risk of falling than other drugs.

A recent study at the Vanderbilt University School of Medicine has shown that nursing home residents who take antidepressants do fall more often than residents who don't take medication for depression. In fact, as the dose increases, so does the risk of falling.

However, the study — which included almost 2,500 people — also compared the rate of falls between SSRIs and tricyclic antidepressants. The results showed they were about the same.

Several medical conditions can also increase your risk of falling. If they apply to you, take extra precautions and ask your doctor for advice.

- ▶ Vision or hearing loss
- ▶ Urinary problems
- ▶ Alzheimer's disease and senility
- ▶ Depression
- ▶ Cancer or other diseases that affect bones
- ▶ Irregular heartbeat
- ▶ Fluctuating blood pressure
- ▶ Arthritis, joint (especially hip) weakness
- ▶ Neurological conditions, strokes, multiple sclerosis, Parkinson's disease

Easy steps to better balance

Losing your balance can be scary. A misstep can lead to a fall and possibly a serious injury. Mental or emotional unbalance can be equally distressing.

Fortunately, you can help yourself maintain balance in all three areas — body, mind, and emotions — with a simple exercise program called tai chi. Tai chi is a "soft" martial art that has been practiced for centuries by millions of Chinese. Today it is growing in popularity with people all around the world.

Karen Sifton teaches tai chi through the continuing education department of the State University of West Georgia. She says anyone can learn it, regardless of their age, size, or athletic ability. Unlike more vigorous forms of exercise that require strength and speed, tai chi emphasizes balanced, flowing movements and inner calm.

"At its heart, it is a superior method of self-improvement," says Sifton. "For the body, it's physical exercise. For the mind, a study in concentration, discipline, and visualization. For the spirit, it's a form of meditation. It's about relaxing into life and enjoying the power that results."

Protects against falls. Every year 30 percent of people over age 65 suffer a fall. And quite a few of these tumbles result in serious injuries.

Whatever your age, the best prevention is exercise that strengthens your muscles and improves your balance. The smooth, low-impact movements of tai chi fit the bill perfectly. And best of all, this gentle activity has been proven to prevent falls.

Dr. Steven Wolf and his associates at the Emory University School of Medicine studied 200 people ages 70 and older. They found that subjects who completed a 15-week tai chi program took about half as many falls as before. The tai chi group also had far fewer falls than other groups who went through high-tech computerized balance training or who received information on preventing falls but no specific training.

Wolf discovered that people in the tai chi group slowed down their normal walking speed and took more deliberate steps. And after the training, fewer participants said they were afraid of falling.

Boosts your all-around health. Tai chi is a relatively inexpensive path to preventing falls and improving your health. Among its advantages:

- ▶ You need no equipment or special clothing.
- ▶ It requires very little space.
- ▶ You can do it indoors or outside.
- ▶ You can practice at home alone or with a group of friends.

Along with developing balance and control, you'll also help your health in other ways. Studies show tai chi improves flexibility, strengthens joints, tones muscles, and even helps the immune system. Doctors find it helpful in treating heart disease, high blood pressure, diabetes, and arthritis. And the best thing is, you'll start seeing these benefits right away.

If you're interested in starting a tai chi program, check with local colleges, recreation centers, fitness clubs, or hospitals for information about classes. With all tai chi has in its favor, it's easy to see why this practice — that balances everything but your checkbook — is becoming more popular with people of all ages.

―――――――

Exercise your way to confidence and control

Mike Ellis, of Bremen Georgia, is a tai chi enthusiast who has reaped the benefits of this ancient martial art. He once described himself as awkward and forgetful. But at age 67 he goes through the tai chi form with the same fluid energy and grace as the younger students in his class.

Ellis makes regular trips to the local VA hospital for cardiac therapy. His nurse practitioner there encourages him to keep up the tai chi practice for his health. But he doesn't have to be prodded.

A long life, he says, doesn't particularly interest him. It's the quality of life that matters. "Tai chi is so relaxing and healthy. I never thought of myself as a high-stress person. But when I realize how relaxed I am now, I know I must have been really stressed."

Studies have shown that people who practice tai chi report less tension, depression, anger, fatigue, and confusion. This comes as no surprise to Ellis' instructor, Karen Sifton. She finds that confidence builds as people discover and extend their physical capabilities and self-awareness. As these improvements carry over into other areas, she says, people lead more fulfilling lives.

According to Ellis, tai chi helps him most by heightening his awareness. "It requires concentration," he says. "And it helps you evaluate your progress in life. You see where you are and how far you have to go, not just physically but mentally, too."

Fibromyalgia

Fight pain with a personal plan

If you suffer from fibromyalgia, you can learn a lot from Dottie Abbott. A petite, delicate-looking woman in her "golden years," she arrives at tai chi class at the University of West Georgia with a lively step and a friendly smile. You'd never guess she had ever been slowed down by any disease.

But about nine years ago, Dottie had coronary artery bypass surgery. She thinks that was the trigger for the onset of fibromyalgia syndrome (FMS). This disorder, which affects muscles, ligaments and tendons, is not life-threatening. But the symptoms, including chronic pain and fatigue, can really make life miserable.

Dottie, however, is living proof that life doesn't have to stop when you have FMS. Although there is no cure, with help and self-discipline, you can work out a plan for managing the symptoms. These are some of the things that work for Dottie.

Get the facts. "If you have fibromyalgia," says Dottie, "the most important thing is to learn all you can about it." This takes away some of the mystery and helps you plan your strategies for dealing with it.

Rita Evans is a licensed clinical social worker who supervises the fibromyalgia self-care program at DeKalb Medical Center in Decatur, Ga. She agrees with Dottie on the importance of being informed.

"This condition is not exactly a disease," she explains. "It is a syndrome — a cluster of symptoms. It's hard to diagnose because there is no definitive test. Doctors have to rule out other causes first, so the average diagnosis takes about two years."

If you have pain you think may be caused by fibromyalgia, Evans suggests you see a doctor who is a rheumatologist. Since they are the experts in this field, you should get a faster diagnosis.

Build a network of support. Dottie thinks family members also need to learn about fibromyalgia. She says living with this condition can be hard on everybody. It requires the kind of patience that only comes when you know what's going on.

"What people with the syndrome need most," says Evans, "is to be heard and understood. They experience real pain, and they need those around them to affirm that they are sane."

Some people get encouragement from a support group. Since it's estimated that FMS affects 6 million Americans, it shouldn't be hard to find one. Evans says an education-based group that focuses on self-discipline is best. Spending a lot of time talking about feelings isn't very helpful with this syndrome.

Keep moving. Dottie says if she doesn't exercise, her muscles knot up, making movement slow and painful. "I know people with FMS who just sit around and suffer," she says. "But you can't do that or you'll be miserable."

When she first started tai chi classes three years ago, Dottie was having a lot of trouble with her balance. The progress was slow at first, but in time she learned to move freely and confidently and rarely has a problem with balance now.

Dottie practices yoga and finds the deep breathing and stretching help her muscles stay loose. In addition, she walks regularly — every day if the weather is nice. And she lifts light weights and gets two therapeutic massages a week.

Give attention to others. Dottie finds she handles pain better if she doesn't just focus on herself. So she keeps mentally involved in activities in her hometown of Carrollton, Ga. She teaches adult literacy classes as a volunteer two mornings a week. And she's on the board of directors of the League of Women Voters.

Stay calm. Stress can trigger fibromyalgia pain, but Dottie has learned to see it coming and side-step it with relaxation. From time to time when she drives into nearby Atlanta to visit her children, she uses the breathwork she learned from yoga and tai chi.

"When I get stuck in traffic," she says, "I just take three deep breaths and relax and let all those other people worry with the frustration. I tell myself everything is just fine."

Get good rest. If you want to stay active in spite of FMS, it's important to get plenty of rest. But that's not easy when you are hurting all over.

Evans says some people find a low dose of an antidepressant — at chronic pain levels, not at clinical depression levels — helps them rest. But Dottie turned down her doctor's offer of drugs. "Everybody handles it differently," she says, "but I think for me exercise takes the place of medication."

"Mild depression often goes with FMS," says Evans. "But touch, exercise, and being with positive people releases endorphins, which relieve depression."

And to round out your self-care plan, Evans recommends eating regular, nutritious meals. As part of an overall healthy lifestyle, these steps, she feels, take the emphasis off FMS symptoms and make it easier to get on with your life.

Foot Pain

Simple ways to conquer heel pain

Heel pain is the most common complaint heard in foot clinics. Some of the causes are arthritis, tendinitis, bursitis, heel spurs, and plantar fasciitis (damage to the rubber band-like tissue on the bottom of your foot). And sometimes heel pain is caused by the choices you make every day. Are you exercising too hard? Do you wear impractical shoes that pinch or rub? Do you stand at your job?

If the pain is severe or accompanied by other symptoms like tingling, numbness, leg cramps, or fever, see your doctor. Otherwise, try these easy, practical tips.

Benefit from some bang-up bargains. You can buy custom-made shoe inserts, called orthoses, and pay anywhere from $300 to $1,000. In some cases, the cost may be necessary. But for less than $50, you can get over-the-counter silicone heel cushions, heel cups, felt heel pads, or arch supports and get the same pain relief. In fact, researchers have found that these inexpensive alternatives are often more effective. It can't hurt to try these simple remedies first and see if you can walk away from foot pain.

Pamper your tootsies. Soaking your feet in warm water for five to 10 minutes will loosen your muscles and soothe your aches. Follow up with a gentle massage, and you'll be in foot heaven.

Practice no-sweat stretches. Stretch the muscles in your calves, ankles, and heels every day. Here are some good exercises to try:

▶ Place a golf ball or a can of frozen fruit juice concentrate on the floor and gently roll your foot over it with light pressure. The frozen juice method gives you the added benefit of an ice massage.

▶ Stand facing a wall. Place your heel on the floor and your toes up on the wall. Push against the wall to gently stretch your heel and the bottom of your foot.

▶ Stand with only the front half of both feet on a step. Hold on to something for balance and gently sink your heels down toward the floor.

Plan a shoe shakedown. Experts say three-fourths of people suffering from heel pain are women, and the reason is as close as their shoe closet.

▶ The most common source of foot misery is the high heel shoe. When wearing "heels," the muscles in your feet, ankles, and calves are placed in an unnatural position, causing tendon damage and joint strain. Don't compromise health for fashion.

▶ Shoes that are flat with thin soles can be just as bad as high heels. They offer no cushioning for your heel or support for your arch.

▶ Unfortunately, shoes do not age gracefully. Take inventory and toss out any worn-out, broken-down shoes. They may be comfortable, but they're not doing your feet any good. Replace them with new shoes that fit well and have good support and padding.

▶ The shoe industry has always assumed that women's feet are just like men's — only smaller. And they have made women's shoes accordingly, smaller versions of men's. However, women everywhere can tell you that this theory is wrong. Men's feet are rectangular, while women's feet are wider at the ball and skinnier at the heel. This makes it difficult to get a good fit. Keep looking until you find a manufacturer suited to your size.

Slim down. If you're overweight, try to lose those extra pounds. They not only place stress on your feet but your other joints as well.

Take two and turn in. For quick pain relief, try an anti-inflammatory, like aspirin or ibuprofen. Then put your feet up for a while and relax.

Get footloose with vitamin C. One health expert recommends applying vitamin C directly on your heel to relieve the discomfort of heel spurs. For this natural remedy, mix water and vitamin C powder until it forms a thick paste. Then spoon some onto a piece of gauze and tape it securely to your heel. Repeat this for several days. The theory is that collagen and elastin from the vitamin C are absorbed through the skin and into the tendon.

Lace away foot pain

If your shoes never fit right, if you are constantly getting blisters, or if you suffer from calluses and bunions, you could pay a lot of money for custom-fitted shoes, or you could try this clever idea that won't cost you a penny. By lacing your shoes in different patterns, you can take a load off your aching feet.

High arches or a sore spot on top of the foot. Skip the set of eyelets closest to the highest part of your foot. You can also feed the laces straight across rather than in a crisscross pattern.

Toe problems. Start the lace in the upper right eyelet. Run the lace down through the bottom left eyelet. Run the lace straight across through the bottom right eyelet. Continue threading the lace diagonally up the shoe until you reach the top. This should help relieve the pressure that causes hammertoes or corns.

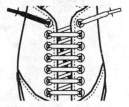

Heel problems. Thread the laces in the normal crisscross pattern, starting at the bottom. At the eyelet that's next to the top, feed the lace through, then feed it through the top eyelet on the same side. Run the lace diagonally down to the eyelet that's next to the top on the opposite side. Follow this pattern on both sides of the shoe. The laces should feed through each other at the top. This lets you tie the shoe snugly without putting too much pressure on the heel.

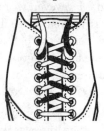

Forgetfulness

Super brain boosters help 'jog' memory

You open the refrigerator door and stand there wondering what you're looking for. Or maybe you go to the grocery store and leave your list at home. You don't recall being so forgetful when you were younger.

Should you worry? Probably not. Lapses in memory are more common with age — so relax. Worry won't help. In fact, stress seems to make memory problems worse.

If you want to increase what your brain retains, try these natural brain boosters.

Vitamin B12. Sardines, chicken livers, tuna, cottage cheese, and sirloin steak, which are rich in vitamin B12, can help restore your short-term memory loss. In a scientific study, people who took vitamin B12 improved their memory within 10 to 27 days. Since vitamin B12 comes only from animal foods, if you are a strict vegetarian, you may not be getting enough.

Folic acid. In another study, people between ages 75 and 96 were tested on their ability to recall words. Those with high levels of vitamin B12 and folic acid (B9) in their blood did better than those with lower levels. Spinach, broccoli, oranges, whole grains, beans, and peas are good sources of folic acid.

Thiamin. Forgetting those things you need to remember can waste time and cause you frustration. Fortunately, memory loss can be restored with another B vitamin — thiamin (B1).

Most people get enough of this vitamin by eating whole grains, seeds, beans, nuts, lean pork, and salmon. Brewer's yeast and wheat germ are even better sources.

Elderly people who don't eat a well-balanced diet are particularly at risk for a thiamin deficiency. If you think you aren't getting enough, a B-complex vitamin should give you enough thiamin and other B vitamins to keep your memory sharp.

Antioxidants. Eating lots of fruits, vegetables, seeds, nuts, and grains helps open the door to your storehouse of memories. These foods contain powerful antioxidants, like vitamin C, vitamin E, beta carotene, and selenium. Research shows as the level of antioxidant nutrients in your blood rises, so does your mental function.

Earlier studies have found that vitamin E helps restore memory loss to people with Alzheimer's. Recently, however, researchers in Austria found that antioxidants in vitamin E, vitamin A, and the carotenoids, like beta carotene, also help older people without Alzheimer's, or any form of dementia, improve their memories.

Other studies show that vitamin C and beta carotene, which changes to vitamin A in the body, help people retain their long-term ability to think, reason, and remember.

Ginkgo. Ginkgo biloba has been used in China and Europe to treat memory loss in older people for hundreds of years. And research shows the older you are the better it works. In one study, this potent herb improved memory by 70 percent for people ages 50 to 70. For those ages 30 to 50, memory increased only 20 percent.

Ginkgo also improves the memory of people with Alzheimer's disease, and the longer they use it, the more it helps. This herb opens up the blood vessels, allowing more blood to get to the brain. And more blood flow means more brain power and better memory.

Ginseng. Ginseng is one of the world's most popular herbs. At least four studies indicate that ginseng can improve memory and concentration. In one study of people ages 50 to 85, memory improved significantly when they took 50 milligrams (mg) of ginseng three times a day for two months. There are a lot of imitators, so look for Asian ginseng. This is the variety that has been studied most. You may find it by the scientific name *Panax ginseng*.

Phosphatidylserine (PS). If you can recall the name of this natural memory booster, you probably don't need more of it. Your body produces this nutrient, a type of fat, from foods you eat. It is found throughout the body, especially in brain cells.

Research shows that PS levels in the brain decline with age. People with age-related memory loss and those with Alzheimer's can benefit by replacing it. You can get it from lecithin, a common food additive, as well as from soy. Supplements are also available.

Sugar. Even though your memory may be sharp for things you've known a long time, there's a tendency to forget new information as you get older. The good news is you may be able to dissolve your forgetfulness with a little sugar. In a study of older people, those who drank lemonade sweetened with sugar did better on memory tests than those who drank lemonade containing saccharin.

But don't rely on sugar as your main memory booster. The calories will mount up too fast. To get sugar more naturally, have a piece of fruit or a glass of orange juice.

Docosahexaenoic acid (DHA). You won't have to worry about the one that got away — the memory, that is — if you eat enough cold-water fish. Experts recommend you eat fatty fish, like salmon, mackerel, and tuna, two or three times a week. This kind of fish contains a lot of DHA, an omega-3 fatty acid, that really does make fish "brain food."

Vegetarians or others who just can't bring themselves to eat fish may want to consider fish oil capsules. But be careful to limit the amount to 3 to 5 grams a day. Fish oil supplements are made from fish skins and livers, which may contain toxic pesticides and other contaminants. Fish oil contains high levels of vitamins A and D, which can also be toxic if you take too much.

Give some of these natural memory boosters a try, and before you know it, you'll be singing, "Thanks for the memories."

Snack your way to a smarter you

It sounds almost too good to be true — junk food that provides you with the extra nutrients you need for better health. While snack foods are still a long way from being nutritional powerhouses, medical science is indeed discovering new ways to make our foods healthier and more beneficial.

"Nutraceuticals" is the fancy name for foods that manufacturers fortify with vitamins, herbs, or other nutrients. This is nothing new — you probably already know that foods such as milk and cereal are fortified with vitamins and minerals. But today, more and more products are being touted as easy and delicious ways to improve your health.

If you want to revive your memory, several companies claim they have the answer. You can just snack on their low-fat cheese curls fortified with ginkgo and reap the benefits of this medicinal herb.

Experts warn that while there's no harm in such snacks, you shouldn't expect to see spectacular results. According to herbal expert Varro Tyler, a typical 1-ounce serving contains about one-tenth of what you'd need to gain any health benefits from herbal additives. To see results, you'd have to eat 10 servings, so even if the snacks are low-fat, the fat and calories can really add up.

Even chewing gum has jumped on the superfood bandwagon. The makers of Brain Gum claim that chewing three pieces of their special gum a day will improve your memory, concentration, and ability to learn. That's because the gum is fortified with a 40 percent concentration of phosphatidylserine (PS), a naturally occurring nutrient that has been shown to have remarkable healing powers in the brain.

Reported to work even better and faster than ginkgo, PS supplements have in many cases successfully reversed declines in mental sharpness that are often associated with aging. Such smart chewing doesn't come cheap, though. Expect to pay about $2 a day for this brain-fixing treat.

Gout

Easy ways to guard against gout

If you're a man over 40 who is a bit overweight and likes his beer, you may someday find yourself with a bad case of gout. This form of arthritis used to be called the "disease of kings" because of its association with rich foods and alcohol. But gout can attack anyone, even women, and once you suffer its agonizing pain, you'll realize just how serious this disease can be.

Gout occurs when you have too much uric acid in your blood. The uric acid forms crystals that lodge in your joints, usually your big toe, and cause inflammation and pain.

You're more likely to get this condition if you are overweight, abuse alcohol, or eat a lot of purine-rich foods. So the most important ways you can help guard against it are to lose weight and make the following diet and lifestyle changes.

Pass by the purines. High-purine foods can cause gout or worsen its symptoms because purines break down to form uric acid.

▶ Most meats are high in purines. You should avoid bacon, turkey, veal, venison, and organ meats such as brains, heart, kidney, and liver. Eat moderate amounts of beef, poultry, ham, and pork. Better sources of protein are tofu and rabbit. Tofu helps your body get rid of uric acid, and rabbit is not only low in purines, it is also low in fat and easy to digest.

▶ Some of your favorite vegetables may be high in purines so eat them sparingly. These include asparagus, beans, cauliflower, lentils, mushrooms, peas, and spinach.

▶ Many fish contain omega-3 fatty acids, which are known to relieve arthritis pain. But seafood can also be loaded with purines. Scientists have proven that the bad effects of the purines in these foods outweigh any benefits you may receive. So if you're at risk for gout, you're better off avoiding anchovies, sardines, herring, trout, codfish, haddock, and shellfish.

Give up the alcohol. Drinking alcohol, especially binge drinking, not only increases your risk of gout, but makes the attacks worse. Beer, in particular, is high in purines. Restrict your use of alcohol, and instead, drink as much water as possible. It will dilute the uric acid in your body and help flush it out of your kidneys.

Beware of drug triggers. In some cases, gout can be caused by thiazide diuretics — "water pills" used to treat high blood pressure. This form of gout usually attacks the hand and knee joints of older women with poor kidney function. If you take this type of drug, and you get severe pain in your hands or knees, ask your doctor to check you for gout.

While there is no cure for gout, prompt diagnosis and treatment will help keep it under control. But by recognizing your risk factors and taking preventive steps now, you may be lucky enough to escape this crippling disease altogether.

Hair Loss

When to be concerned about hair loss

If you are a woman who enjoys brushing her hair, you may not mind the little bit that comes out in the brush. But if you are losing more of your "crowning glory" than usual, you are likely to be concerned.

Some hair shedding is normal. Your hair has a cycle of growth, rest, and regrowth. The average person loses 100 to 125 hairs a day as some in the resting stage fall out, making way for the new.

Heavier hair loss, however, can be more serious. Fortunately, in most cases the loss is temporary. But knowing the reasons your hair is coming out can put your mind at rest or alert you to the need for treatment.

Get to the root of your hair loss. Dr. Amy McMichael of Wake Forest University is a dermatologist specializing in skin, nail, and hair problems. She points out one of the most common causes of hair loss — telogen effluvium, or resting hair loss. "All women have it at some time. It probably happens in men, too. They just don't notice," says McMichael.

This type of hair loss usually occurs after a stressful situation causes more hair than usual to go into the resting phase of the growth cycle. Three to six months later, shedding becomes noticeable. These are some stressors that may trigger this condition.

- ▶ **Illness or emotional stress.** You may notice shedding following an injury, infection, fever, surgery, or the loss of a loved one.

- ▶ **Hormone changes.** During pregnancy hair often gets thicker, but after the birth of the baby, you may start losing your locks.

▶ **Rapid weight loss.** Reducing too much or too quickly from extremely low-calorie diets can make your hair fall out. And supplements, especially those high in vitamin A, may make the problem worse. A balanced diet, on the other hand, promotes healthy hair growth.

▶ **Anemia and thyroid problems.** You may need a simple blood test to determine if you need more iron or thyroid hormones.

▶ **Medications.** Likely culprits are antidepressants, birth control pills, blood thinners, and gout medicine. Check with your doctor if you suspect this might be the cause of your hair loss. Perhaps you can take a different medication that doesn't have this undesirable side effect.

This kind of hair shedding rarely causes baldness. Usually, no more than 50 percent of your hair falls out. When the stress has passed, your hair's normal growth cycle can begin again. But it does take a while to get back to your normal thickness and possibly longer to reach its former length.

McMichael says people frequently go to a dermatologist at the height of their hair loss. "They've probably been having it for a while but just haven't noticed it being severe enough to worry about it. So we usually see people after around three to six months," she says.

"After another three months, it tapers off. Three more months and it begins to regrow." She suggests you give it a year before you worry that you are having some other problem.

Get professional help. Some conditions require more than eliminating stress and waiting patiently for regrowth. If shedding doesn't slow down, you might want to see a dermatologist. You may need help with these as well:

▶ **Unhealthy scalp conditions.** "Pain, itching, drainage, excessive flaking, or redness in your scalp are signs to seek out a dermatologist," says McMichael. "You need the right person to evaluate you and try to integrate that into your medical care."

- ► **Fallout due to an illness.** Hair loss may accompany a disease like diabetes, lupus, or rheumatoid arthritis. Your regular doctor may treat your hair loss or refer you to a dermatologist.

- ► **Thinning related to hormone changes.** Both men and women get the condition known as male-pattern or female-pattern baldness. Women usually experience thinning, not baldness, over the top of the scalp. This condition seems to be hereditary, but because it is usually hormone related, you may find it more of a problem after menopause.

Get treatment for fallout. Today's options for treating hair loss include oral medications, topical creams, corticosteroid injections, and hair transplants. Although many of the ointments and medications on the market have been FDA approved only for men, there are some that can be helpful to women.

In some cases, however, females may experience side effects like skin irritations and increased facial hair. So let your dermatologist advise you about the use of these products.

"There are a lot of unanswered questions about hair loss in women," says McMichael. "But we are increasing our awareness every day with research.

Protect your 'mane' feature

Your hair, like that of many women, may be what makes you stand out in a crowd. Unfortunately, you may be damaging your beautiful tresses with products and practices that cause weathering, or breakage. That may contribute to hair loss. Dermatologist Amy McMichael offers these suggestions for better hair care.

Stop practices that damage hair. Hot rollers, curling irons, harsh chemicals, hot oil treatments, tight braids — all these can be stressful to your scalp. If you don't correct the damage they do before scarring occurs, hair loss can be permanent, McMichael says.

"You may have learned them from your mother, grandmother, an aunt, or maybe even a hairdresser — but they may not be correct." She suggests you save the heavy styling for special occasions.

Minimize breakage with a little pampering. McMichael recommends using moisturizing shampoos and conditioners. And she suggests getting hair trimmed every six-to-eight weeks. Hair stylists, she notes, are often the first to notice signs of hair loss and bald spots.

Trust your hair to an expert. If you use two or more hair treatments — such as color and a perm — see a qualified hair stylist, McMichael advises. Don't try to do it yourself. Although some people manage it without harmful effects, she says most people aren't so lucky.

Be wary of advertisers' promises. McMichael warns that not all advertised products live up to their claims, especially those over-the-counter potions that promise you'll grow hair faster and longer.

"There is nothing known to man that can increase the rate of growth," she says. "There are things that can improve hair structure so it doesn't break off and things that can be done to allow hair to be healthier. But nothing that will increase the rate or the set length your hair is going to be."

A 'scents'ible way to make hair grow

Since ancient times, people have added fragrance to their hair with herbs and spices. But research now finds that oils from some aromatic plants may do more than add a pleasant smell to your tresses — they may also hold the key to replacing lost locks.

In Scotland, researchers tested aromatherapy on people with alopecia areata, a condition that causes hair to come out in patches. Half of those in the study massaged thyme, rosemary, lavender, and cedarwood essential oils, mixed with "carrier" oils, into their scalps each day.

The other half massaged their scalps daily with just the carrier oils, grapeseed and jojoba. Neither group knew which mixture they were using, but all followed the same directions.

After seven months, those using the mixture with the essential oils had an amazing 44 percent improvement in hair growth. The other group improved as well, but only by 15 percent. So it was clear to the researchers that the scalp massages didn't work most of the magic. At least one of the essential oils stimulated hair growth.

In addition, results of this aromatherapy trial showed that essential oils regrow hair as well or better than the usual treatments for alopecia areata. And they are also safer. The conventional treatments can have undesirable side effects.

Even if you don't have a problem with hair loss, you might enjoy a soothing aromatic scalp massage. Here's the recipe the researchers used:

- ▶ Essential oils:
  Thyme vulgaris — 2 drops (88 mg)
  Lavandula agustifolia — 3 drops (108 mg)
  Rosmarinus officinalis — 3 drops (114 mg)
  Cedrus atlantica — 2 drops (94 mg)

- ▶ Carrier oils:
  jojoba — 3 mL
  grapeseed — 20 mL

Blend oils together and massage into your scalp for two minutes each night. Wrap your head in a warm towel to help the skin absorb the oils.

Look for essential oils at herb shops, health food stores, and drugstores.

Headaches

18 ways to halt headache pain fast

Most headaches are caused by tension. You know the feeling — a dull, constant ache that begins on both sides of your head. It can feel like a headband is squeezing tighter and tighter around your temples and the back of your skull.

What you really need is to get rid of all the tension in your life, but that's just not possible. So instead, form a plan of action that includes these headache-fighting tips.

Take five. Just a few minutes of rest in a dark, quiet room may be all you need to relax and ease your tensions away.

Heat it up. Place a slightly damp washcloth in the microwave and zap it until it's just warm to the touch — be careful not to get it too hot. Lay down and place it on your forehead.

Cool it down. Place an ice pack or frozen gel pack on the back of your head or neck.

Wash pain down the drain. Take a long, relaxing bath or hot steamy shower, and feel your tense muscles loosen up.

Get relief over the counter. Ibuprofen, acetaminophen, or aspirin are all good, safe pain-relievers. For them to work best, remember to take them sparingly — not every day — and at the first sign of a headache.

Pinch an inch. Use accupressure on three points above each eyebrow. Gently pinch about an inch of skin close to the bridge of your nose, then over the center of your eye, and again at the outermost point of your eyebrow.

Breathe deeply. Relax your shoulder and neck muscles, and breathe in from your belly. (See the *Stress* chapter for information on deep breathing exercises.)

Sit up straight. Placing your body in awkward positions puts a strain on your spine and neck muscles and can lead to headaches.

Grab some magic fingers. There's nothing like a soothing scalp massage to knead away pain and tension. Go to a professional, or ask a friend to help out. Teach your spouse or try giving one to yourself. Many shampooers at salons make this part of their regular hair care service.

Know your no-no's. Many headaches are brought on by specific things, especially foods. Keep a diary, noting what triggers your head pain, and learn to avoid these.

Don't be a caffeine fiend. If you usually drink coffee or caffeinated sodas, stopping suddenly can cause a withdrawal headache. On the other hand, if you start drinking more than usual, your blood vessels will constrict and give you a headache. If you must have caffeine, try to identify a safe amount for yourself, and stick with it.

Put out the fire. Stop smoking. Just do it.

Rethink the drink. Some people don't have to empty the bottle to get a king-size hangover — even an occasional glass of wine can bring on a pounding head. Choose your beverages wisely.

Go for high energy. Get regular exercise, like swimming, cycling, and walking. This keeps your blood flowing and your muscles limber, and takes your mind off your headache.

Turn in on time. Your brain and your body need the right amount of sleep on a regular basis in order to function well and fight off stress.

Banish the blues. If you suffer from depression headaches, which can hit first thing in the morning, get help from your doctor, a counselor, or even a friend.

Learn from the pros. Relaxation therapy and biofeedback are two treatments you can learn from professionals that will help you control pain.

Get by with a little help from your friends. Join a headache support group where you can share information and remedies. Or begin your own.

Alternative answers to migraine pain

Migraines can be the most disabling of all headaches. Not only do you experience excruciating head pain, you may suffer nausea and vomiting; sensitivity to light, sound and odors; and visual disturbances such as jagged or flashing lights. Attacks can last days or even weeks and force you to stay in bed until you recover. If migraines are part of your life, all you want is relief. Here are some alternative forms of treatment that just might work for you.

Try an age-old remedy. If you had lived a few hundred years ago, you might have picked a handful of feverfew leaves, crushed them, sweetened them with honey, and used them to bring down a fever. Today, researchers have found this herb may be just as helpful in preventing migraine pain. Several studies testing feverfew on migraine sufferers have shown it can reduce the number of migraine attacks and ease even severe symptoms.

You can buy feverfew preparations at a health or nutrition store. Check the label to be sure it contains at least 0.2 percent parthenolide. That's the main ingredient that reduces pain and causes the migraines to come less often.

Sniff your migraine away. Fifty chronic headache patients tried doing just that in a study at the Smell and Taste Treatment and Research Foundation in Chicago. Since some odors like perfumes, food, or cigarette smoke seem to trigger migraines, experts wanted to find out if odors could also relieve migraine pain.

They tested the scent of green apples and found that some migraine sufferers responded well while others didn't. The deciding factor seemed to be how much they liked the odor. Researchers believe you should find a scent that is pleasing to you or that you associate with pleasant memories. These are more likely to reduce your headache pain.

Mind your Cs and Ds. Here's another reason to get more calcium and vitamin D — they could help relieve your migraine pain.

In two small studies, women with low levels of vitamin D who suffered from migraines had fewer attacks and less severe symptoms when they took calcium and vitamin D supplements.

Manage better with magnesium. Many people who suffer from migraines have very little of this mineral in their bodies. Researchers aren't sure if the low levels actually cause you to have migraines or if people with low levels are simply more likely to have migraines.

Some migraine sufferers respond well to taking magnesium supplements — they have fewer attacks and less pain. If you want to try it, the recommended dietary allowance is between 320 and 420 milligrams (mg) per day. Don't take more than 350 mg/day in supplement form, or you may experience dangerous side effects.

Beware: Supplement may be contaminated

If you're searching for a natural cure to your headache pain, be careful. One supplement recommended for migraines may be contaminated with a dangerous substance.

The amino acid 5-HTP (hydroxy-L-tryptophan) is a popular dietary supplement touted as a natural way to overcome depression, obesity, and insomnia. It has also been recommended as an effective migraine cure.

But researchers at the Mayo Clinic found that samples of 5-HTP contained impurities that could be harmful. Food and Drug Administration (FDA) scientists confirmed those findings.

One of the impurities, known as "peak X," was identified in a case of eosinophilia myalgia syndrome (EMS) associated with 5-HTP in 1991. The FDA banned a related supplement, L-tryptophan, in 1989 after an epidemic of EMS illnesses and deaths. Impurities similar to peak X were implicated in the outbreak.

Researchers did not find a high level of peak X in the 5-HTP samples they examined. But no one knows for sure how much of the contaminant is safe, and if you take large doses of the supplement, you could end up seriously ill.

You need to be extra careful when dealing with "natural" supplements because they do not require FDA approval like prescription drugs and over-the-counter medications. If you have questions about 5-HTP or any other supplement, talk to your doctor.

Stop the food-headache cycle

You are what you eat. It's not just an old saying — science has proven that foods make a huge impact on your health and well-being. And if you suffer from chronic headaches, what you are eating could be the cause of your pain. Here are some of the most common headache triggers.

Food additives. Substances added to processed foods to preserve them and add flavor may add more than you bargained for.

▶ **Aspartame** is an artificial sweetener that you can add to foods or drinks yourself or buy already in low-calorie foods and diet drinks. Nutrasweet and Equal are two of the brand names. Some studies link aspartame with migraine headaches, and others do not.

▶ **Monosodium glutamate (MSG)** is a flavor enhancer often reported by migraine sufferers as a headache trigger. Although once it was associated mainly with Chinese food, it is also used in Accent, meat tenderizers, canned meat and fish, and packaged and prepared foods. The FDA requires MSG to be listed as an ingredient on food labels.

▶ **Sodium nitrite** is used in processed meats like hot dogs, turkey, ham, and sausage and can cause headaches in some people.

Alcohol. Why does alcohol give you a headache? Because of chemicals called congeners and histamines. Congeners give a special aroma and flavor to each type of alcohol. Red wine and beer contain the highest amounts, and since these drinks are most often associated with headaches, researchers believe there is some connection.

Histamines are found naturally in your body and in certain foods. But if you are histamine intolerant, your system can't break down these substances properly. One result may be that blood vessels in your brain expand, causing headache pain.

Histamines are found in all types of wine, but red can have up to 200 times more than white. They are also in beer, sardines, anchovies, ripened cheeses, hard-cured sausages like pepperoni and salami, and pickled vegetables. If you think you are histamine intolerant, talk to your doctor about going on a histamine-free diet.

Cold foods. A dish of ice cream on a hot summer day looks pretty inviting. But after a few bites, a sudden sharp pain strikes in the middle of your forehead. It's the attack of an ice cream headache.

Eating or drinking very cold foods and beverages can cause stabbing head pain, but according to a report in the *British Medical Journal,* ice cream is the most common cause. The pain is usually brief, but intense — peaking in 30 to 60 seconds and fading quickly, although in some cases it can last up to five minutes.

You don't have to give up ice cream to avoid a "brain freeze." Just eat slowly, and try not to let the frozen treat touch the back of the roof of your mouth.

Tyramine. This substance can expand blood vessels in the brain, causing headache pain. It's found in lima beans, fava beans, snow peas, freshly-baked yeast breads or cakes, wine, beer, liver, including paté, and most cheeses.

If you take an MAO inhibitor for depression, you may get a severe headache when you eat certain tyramine-rich foods, like cheese. If you're on this type of medication, see if avoiding these foods makes a difference in how often you get headaches.

Caffeine. If you don't get your morning cup of coffee, your head may begin to pound. That's the first sign of caffeine withdrawal. Many people forget that caffeine is a drug. The more you drink, the more your body comes to depend on it. When you finally get that

first can of cola, cup of tea, or mug of coffee, your withdrawal symptoms go away. No more headache. That is, until tomorrow.

If you don't like being dependent on caffeine, try limiting yourself to only eight ounces a day — the amount recommended by the
National Headache Foundation. If you drink more than that now, it's
best to cut back gradually to avoid headaches.

Caffeine can be helpful in some instances though. Some of the
most effective headache medications contain caffeine as an ingredient. And some migraine sufferers swear by a cup or two of strong tea
or coffee at the onset of a headache to prevent or ease the pain.

Reactions to different foods can vary from one person to another. Even such common foods as sour cream, peanut butter, sour-
dough bread, pizza, bananas, and raisins can give some people a
headache. Keep a diary of what you eat and when your head hurts,
and you should be able to pinpoint your own triggers.

Hearing Loss

16 strategies to improve your hearing

Your ears are not like other parts of your body. Working them harder won't make them stronger. The delicate mechanisms that make up your inner ear are very sensitive. You can damage your hearing gradually doing ordinary, everyday activities without knowing you're doing any harm.

While you can't isolate yourself completely from harsh noises, there are steps you can take to minimize your exposure — and there are ways to cope with hearing loss.

Quiet your world. The more noise you cut from your day, the better it is for your ears. Try reducing noise from appliances, printers, and typewriters by placing them on rubber mats. Block out street and other outside noise with drapes, fabric wall hangings, and double-paned windows. The best absorber of indoor noise is a plush carpet.

Insulate your ears. If you're going to be working at a loud task, prepare beforehand. Using power tools, riding motorcycles or snow-mobiles, and discharging firearms are all common activities loud enough to cause serious damage to your ears over time. To prevent this, wear foam earplugs. They are inexpensive, and you can buy them at hardware or discount stores.

Stop abusing noise. A lot of people use noise to cover noise, which only makes things harder on your delicate ears. If a loud noise is bothering you, don't turn up the TV or stereo to drown it out. Instead, see if there's anything you can do to avoid the noise.

Get used to quiet. Try lowering the volume on your radio, TV, and headset. People often listen at a certain volume more out of habit than necessity. If someone standing nearby can hear sounds coming from your headphones, you've got them turned up too loud. Try keeping the noise in your home to a bare minimum.

Give them rest. Your ears need time to recover, especially after a really loud day. Giving them a few hours of low-noise time can help them recuperate from a day's worth of wear and tear.

Don't strain. Extreme physical stress can raise the level of pressure in your ears to a dangerous level and cause damage to your hearing. Use extra caution when lifting heavy objects or exerting yourself in any way.

Exercise regularly. Add hearing to the list of things exercise helps. Exercise improves the circulation of blood to your inner ear where it helps keep hearing mechanisms, such as your sound-detecting hair cells, in good working order.

Ditch the wax. If you think your hearing is going, check your earwax. Cleaning out your ears can sometimes clear up your hearing. To learn the best ways to do it, see *Safest ways to clean your ears*.

Check your medicine. Some drugs can cause or contribute to hearing loss. Aspirin, furosemide, neomycin, and gentamicin are common culprits. If you take any of these drugs, have your hearing checked regularly.

Talk in corners. Standing in a corner puts two surfaces behind you to reflect sound and make it easier to hear. It creates the same effect as cupping your hand over your ear — it helps to catch the sound and direct it where it's needed.

Speak up. If you can't hear someone, ask them to speak in a deeper tone of voice. When hearing damage occurs, high-pitched noises are among the first you lose. Lower tones are easier to pick up.

Wear a hearing aid. Hearing aids can work wonders for you, and they are getting better and more affordable every day. Be sure to have yours fitted by a doctor. Although dealers know their product, only a doctor can examine you, find out the cause of your hearing loss, and suggest alternative treatments.

Tune in to the latest technology. If your hearing loss is permanent, but not total, there are many things you can do around the house to make it easier to hear. Some of the helpers available are amplifiers for your phone, your TV, and VCR. Just about anything that makes noise can be retooled to make the noise louder.

Protect yourself at home. For safety's sake, make sure every alarm in your home is loud enough to alert you. Test the buzzer on your doorbell, your oven, security system, smoke detectors, and the ring of your telephone. If you can't hear these sounds, they can be replaced or supplemented with flashing lights.

Closed captioning, which allows you to read along with what's being said on screen, is available on most new televisions. The technology of TDD (Telecommunication Device for the Deaf) helps make phone calls easier. More and more companies and agencies are getting TDD lines to accommodate the needs of the hearing impaired.

Get tested for free. For a quick, free test of your hearing, call Dial a Hearing Test at 1-800-222-EARS (3277). They'll give you a local number you can call to take a two-minute hearing test over the phone.

Learn the facts. To learn more about what options and opportunities are available to people with hearing problems, contact one of the organizations listed here.

National Association of the Deaf
Phone: (301) 587-1788
TTY: (301) 587-1789

National Information Center on Deafness
Phone: 800-241-1044
TTY: 800-241-1055

Alexander Graham Bell Association for the Deaf
Phone: (202) 337-5220
TTY: (202) 337-5221

Safest ways to clean your ears

If you're like most people, earwax is something you never think about, but maybe you should. This yellowish secretion protects your inner ear from potentially damaging things, like sand, dirt, and insects.

But too much earwax can make hearing difficult. In extreme cases, it can block the ear canal. Having very hairy or narrow ears can make the problem even worse.

If you're having trouble with earwax, follow this advice from the experts.

Toss aside the cotton swabs. Did your mother ever tell you not to stick anything smaller than your elbow in your ear? She was right. Trying to pick at earwax with your fingers, tweezers, or other sharp objects could cause serious injury. Even cotton swabs are a no-no. Doctors say a swab is more likely to push the wax deeper into your ear.

Flush it away. Fill a bowl or bathroom sink with warm water. Using a rubber ball syringe, turn your head to one side and flush one ear at a time with water, dropping the water in gently. Never apply more than just the slightest bit of pressure. Remember, you're trying to soften the wax, not blast it out.

Try a drop of oil. If warm water hasn't done the trick, try a different approach. Use an eyedropper to place a couple of drops of oil — baby, vegetable, or mineral — into your ear. Hold it in with a cotton ball for a few minutes, then wipe away the excess. Over a day or two, the oil should start to break up the wax. You can also use this technique with hydrogen peroxide, glycerin, or a warm water and vinegar solution.

Chomp down on buildup. Your body's natural defense against earwax buildup isn't an active pinkie finger — it's chewing. The chewing motion of your teeth and jaw actually breaks up earwax and keeps your ear canal in good working order. People who don't chew their food well often have trouble with earwax.

Cut back on fat. If you need another reason to cut the fat out of your diet, here it is. Research has shown that saturated fat, found mostly in foods of animal origin, causes your ears to produce too much earwax. So take it easy on your hearing while you take it easy on your heart — cut back on saturated fat.

Combat hearing loss with vitamins

If you think your hearing is mostly affected by external things, like loud noises, you wouldn't be all wrong. Your ears are very sensitive to sounds and vibrations, and they can easily be damaged.

But hearing loss can also come from the inside, especially if you're deficient in these vitamins.

Vitamin A. Studies show when you don't get enough vitamin A, your ears become extra sensitive to sound. This doesn't mean you hear better, you just hear louder. This intensified noise increases your risk of severe ear damage.

Vitamin A is found in many foods. Egg yolks, butter, and liver are good sources. For a lighter twist, get your vitamin A from oranges, limes, cantaloupe, prunes, and pineapple.

Fish are a good source of vitamin A, but salmon, mackerel, and tuna are especially high in this important nutrient. Fish are also high in vitamin D, which helps prevent bone loss and may help strengthen the bones in the ear's hearing mechanism. That could mean sharper hearing as you get older.

Vitamin B12 and folic acid. Most people think getting a little hard of hearing is a natural part of aging. Recent research suggests this might not be the case. A study at the University of Georgia revealed that women over age 60 who had hearing loss also had lower blood levels of vitamin B12 and folic acid.

Vitamin B12 and folic acid work together to maintain blood flow and to keep your nervous system in good working order. Some researchers think not enough blood flowing to the inner ear can affect the electrical impulses from the ear to the brain. This could cause hearing loss.

Liver, sardines, crab, salmon, beef, and cottage cheese are excellent sources of vitamin B12. If you want more folic acid, eat oranges, avocado, papaya, liver, spinach, pinto beans, lentils, asparagus, and beets.

Although these vitamins play a vital role in preserving your hearing, they won't reverse hearing damage you already have.

Can a pill cure deafness?

What if taking a pill could restore your hearing? Strangely enough, for certain types of hearing loss, it's possible.

Researchers have found that exposure to intense noise causes increased free radical activity in the sensory hair cells of your inner ear. These free radicals attack the hair cells and can damage or destroy them, resulting in hearing loss or deafness.

By building up the level of certain antioxidants by using an antioxidant-enhancing drug before or shortly after exposure to damaging noise, doctors have been able to prevent and even reverse some of the damage. The antioxidant drug essentially takes on the destructive free radicals and keeps them from damaging your ears.

Scientists have also learned that magnesium is vital to hearing. The more you are exposed to loud noise, the more you are drained of your magnesium, and the more susceptible to damage your ears become.

One study measured the hearing of 320 soldiers in training under extreme noise conditions over two months. Half the soldiers took 700 milligrams (mg) of magnesium a day, about twice the RDA, and the other half didn't. Those who took the magnesium ended up with about half the hearing loss of the others.

While the antioxidant-enhancing drug is not yet available to the public, some experts believe preventive and healing pills for treating hearing loss are no more than a year or two away.

How to break-in a new hearing aid

Hearing aids have changed thousands of lives for the better but getting used to one isn't exactly easy. The awkward process of breaking-in a hearing aid is described by some professionals as "re-learning" how to hear. This is because you are forced to use skills you probably haven't used in years.

These simple suggestions can make the transition go more smoothly and pleasantly.

▶ **Be patient with yourself.** Many noises will sound more shrill than you are used to because your ears can now pick up on higher frequencies than before. For this reason, a lot of things won't sound the same as before, but you'll soon learn to recognize the new sounds.

▶ **Know your surroundings.** Some environments will be easier to hear in than others. Noise in rooms with lots of hard surfaces and busy activity will be louder than rooms with lots of sound absorbers, like sofas and carpeting. Knowing where you can hear best will help you make the most of your new ability.

▶ **Learn how to use it.** Have your doctor show you how to use your hearing aid. Then you'll be comfortable adjusting and maintaining it. When making adjustments, do so gradually. You'll soon learn what settings work best for certain situations.

▶ **Take things slowly.** Don't start off wearing your hearing aid 24 hours a day. Take your time and build up slowly. You'll eventually get used to it. At first, you may have a feeling of fullness in your ears or think your voice sounds hollow. Some people feel like they have a head cold. Strangely enough, these are all normal. And if it seems like too much of a hassle to put up with, keep in mind you're getting your hearing back. That ought to put a smile on your face.

Heart Disease

6 ways to fight heart disease from the kitchen

Atherosclerosis occurs when cholesterol, fat, and other substances in your blood build up in the walls of your arteries, forming plaque. Plaque can clog or completely block arteries, cutting off blood flow to your heart or brain. That's when you have a heart attack or stroke.

Too much cholesterol and triglycerides — types of fat — in the blood, high blood pressure, and smoking cause the most damage to your arteries. Other risk factors for atherosclerosis include diabetes, a family history of the condition, stress, obesity, and an inactive lifestyle. Men, in general, are at greater risk, as are people who have an "apple" body shape — with the fat gathering at the belly rather than the hips and thighs.

You can fight atherosclerosis by making good food choices. Cut back on saturated fat and cholesterol from meat and whole-milk dairy products, and look for the following foods that lower cholesterol, bring down blood pressure, and keep your blood flowing smoothly.

Fiber. During the course of a day, you should eat about 25 to 35 grams of fiber. If you do, you'll boost your general health and give atherosclerosis quite a battle.

Certain types of soluble fiber, such as the kind in oats, barley, apples, and other fruits, shrink your cholesterol levels. It works by slowing down your food as it passes through your stomach and small intestine so your "good" cholesterol has more time to take cholesterol to your liver and out of your body. Eating more than 25 grams of fiber every day might also cut your risk of developing high blood pressure by 25 percent.

Fiber comes with an added bonus — it fills you up. After a fiber-rich meal, you feel full, so you're less likely to overeat and put on unwanted pounds. Because being overweight increases your risk of atherosclerosis and other heart problems, eating fiber could be part of an effective strategy to guard your arteries.

You'll find fiber in fruits, vegetables, and whole-grain breads and cereals.

Antioxidants. As your body processes the oxygen you breathe in, it also produces chemicals called free radicals. These are molecules that are unstable because they lack an electron. They travel through your body trying to steal electrons from healthy cells. When they succeed, they leave the cell irreversibly damaged. Over time, they can cause so much damage that your body becomes weak and more likely to fall prey to cancer and heart disease. This cell damage is called oxidation.

Luckily, your body produces antioxidants which neutralize free radicals — a sort of natural "fountain of youth." But as you get older, your body's production of antioxidants slows down. Fortunately, you can get antioxidants from your diet.

Vitamin C, vitamin E, and beta carotene are antioxidants. Peppers, oranges, strawberries, cantaloupe, and broccoli give you vitamin C, while carrots, sweet potatoes, spinach, mangoes, and collard greens are full of beta carotene. Sources of vitamin E include wheat germ, nuts, seeds, and vegetable oils.

While you munch on those fruits and vegetables, you'll get the added benefit of antioxidant substances called flavonoids. Resveratrol in grapes, anthocyanins in cranberry juice, and quercetin in onions, apples, and tea are some of the flavonoids that help your heart and arteries.

Fish. Reel in a big, fat fish and wriggle off the hook of atherosclerosis. Omega-3 fatty acids, the polyunsaturated kinds found in fatty fish like tuna, mackerel, and salmon, protect your arteries from damage.

First, omega-3 takes out triglycerides, the fats that build up on your artery walls. It also stops your blood's platelets from clumping together. That way, your blood remains smooth instead of sticky. Sticky blood can clot and block blood flow. Lastly, omega-3 might lower blood pressure.

No wonder so many studies show that eating fish can reduce your risk of heart disease. The American Heart Association recommends eating at least two fish meals a week.

You can find a form of omega-3 called alpha-linolenic acid in walnuts, which lower cholesterol. Other sources of omega-3 include flaxseed, wheat germ, and some green, leafy vegetables, like kale, spinach, and arugula.

Garlic. Anything fish can do garlic does, too. The sulfur compounds in this amazing herb not only lower cholesterol and triglycerides, but they also go after only the LDL or "bad" cholesterol and leave the HDL or "good" cholesterol alone.

Garlic can also lower blood pressure so your arteries don't take as much of a pounding. Thanks to a substance called ajoene, garlic keeps your blood from clumping and clotting. One study even showed garlic helps your aorta, the body's main artery, remain elastic as you age.

Experts recommend getting 4 grams of garlic — about one clove — into your diet each day.

Monounsaturated fat. To keep your blood running smoothly, maybe you need an oil change. Olive oil, the main source of fat in the heart-healthy Mediterranean diet, has mostly monounsaturated fat. This type of fat slashes the "bad" cholesterol without harming the "good" cholesterol. It also prevents clotting, giving your arteries even more protection. Like fiber, monounsaturated fat also fills you up so you're less likely to overeat.

Think about switching from soybean or corn oil to olive oil. After all, the Greeks — even while enjoying a rather high-fat diet — rarely develop atherosclerosis.

Besides olive oil, sources of monounsaturated fat include avocados, nuts, and canola oil.

Ginger. Make your dinner a little bit tastier and your arteries a little bit healthier with this ancient spice. Ginger contains phytochemicals called gingerol and shogaol, which give it its antioxidant power.

Animal studies show ginger not only lowers LDL cholesterol and triglycerides, it also prevents LDL oxidation. On top of that, ginger also keeps your blood from clotting by reducing the stickiness of your platelets.

New discovery: How your heart helps itself

Here's another good reason to exercise — all that huffing and puffing makes your heart create a protein that may protect it from permanent damage if you have a heart attack. And researchers say you only have to exercise three days to reap the benefits.

Although recent medical studies have tested animals, scientists believe the same thing occurs in humans. They found that a protein, called Heat Shock Protein (HSP) 72, protects the cells of the heart from dying from the stress of an attack.

Once the cells die, they're gone forever, so if you can keep them alive, you have a better chance of surviving a heart attack. Exercise is the key — it's long been known to protect your heart, but researchers now think this stress protein plays a large role in that protection.

All you have to do is exercise three to five days to make enough of the protein to safeguard your heart. But you lose your reserves fairly quickly, so you do need to keep up your exercise routine.

That's why it's never too late to get up and get moving. With less than a week's worth of walking, jogging, or cycling, you can give yourself a stronger, healthier heart.

Safeguard your heart from these hidden dangers

The earthquake hit Jan. 17, 1995, 5:46 a.m. Japan time. For the next four weeks, the number of reported heart attacks more than tripled within the area of the quake. Similar increases were seen after quakes in Greece, Australia, and California.

These may be scary statistics, but experts say natural disasters are only one of many hidden heart attack triggers — and probably the one you least have to worry about. The way you talk to your kids, how seriously you take your job, and even the weather can spell even bigger trouble.

End emotional emergencies. Cartoon characters with steam coming out of their ears, eyes popping from their heads, and faces red as fire engines may be too close to the truth to be funny. Experts have proven that any burst of emotion, whether it's anger, fear, or anxiety, can send your blood pressure through the roof and your heart dangerously close to a life-threatening seizure.

The answer? Relax, control your emotions, and avoid conflict. A German study found that sometimes it's better to let others run the show once in a while. Being passive in certain situations and letting go of some responsibilities could mean lower heart rate and blood pressure.

Work smart, not long. Are you loyal, dedicated, hard-working? These are all wonderful qualities on the job. They could mean increased production, promotions, or higher pay. However, they could also mean a heart attack.

A study in Japan found that longer than average workdays and lengthy commutes greatly increase work tension. Work tension increases blood pressure. And high blood pressure is an important heart attack risk factor. In fact, skyrocketing blood pressure is as bad for your heart as gaining 50 pounds or aging 25 years. So slow down and take the stress off your heart and the strain off your health.

Be aware of job risks. Can you guess which industry hides a secret heart danger? Power companies. Scientists at the Midwest Research Institute collected health information from 140,000 electric-utility workers over a 38-year period. They found a disturbingly high number of heart-rhythm-related deaths.

Linemen and power-plant operators are exposed to strong levels of electromagnetic fields (EMFs), the invisible flow of magnetic energy that's produced by any electric current. The theory is that high-level EMFs cause damaging changes in heart rate — enough to make you up to three times as likely to die of heart problems as your colleagues in other professions.

One argument against this theory is that workers in certain trades are more apt to smoke, drink, and eat a high-fat diet. This heart-risky lifestyle may contribute more to heart disease than exposure to EMFs. Nevertheless, if you work around magnetic fields, you should pay attention to any dramatic changes in your heart rate, and talk to your doctor if you have concerns.

Watch out for winter woes. Better start getting in shape for next winter — especially if you've got some snow shoveling to look forward to. Statistics show that the number of heart attacks peaks in mid-winter. It's not so much the temperature or the shoveling that poses a danger to your heart, it's being out of shape when you find yourself up to your windowsills in the white stuff.

Unusual physical activity like snow shoveling puts an unexpected strain on your heart and even your arteries, increasing the likelihood that plaque will rupture and cause a heart attack. In addition, many people let their immune system pretty much fend for itself, forgetting that winter is prime cold and flu season. A weakened body is more vulnerable to heart attack than a strong one.

Eat right, take a multivitamin, and find time for regular, moderate exercise year-round. This protects your heart by slowly building up strength and endurance. Then when you have to do something strenuous, it's not such a surprise to your body.

Technology may mean trouble for your ticker

Keep your cell phone to your ear, and don't loiter at store entrances. Are these part of the modern code of behavior? No, they're safety rules for people with pacemakers. Experts have found acoustomagnetic fields, like those from cell phones and retail anti-shoplifting gates, can interfere with cardiac pacemakers.

Don't worry, you don't have to give up the modern convenience of a cell phone, but if you use one, don't carry it in a breast pocket. Having an activated phone positioned over your heart may cause a problem with your pacemaker.

And finding a great sale might make your heart go pitter-patter, but one woman with a pacemaker suffered dizziness, nausea and palpitations simply by standing at a store entrance, directly within its electronic antitheft system. Stores will admit that many people have had similar reactions.

You'll be fine, however, if you don't linger in the entrance. Just walk quickly through the security field.

Protect your heart from 'the big chill'

You've heard the old proverb, "It's an ill wind that blows nobody good." This may be truer than you think, particularly if you suffer from heart disease. The American Heart Association has found evidence that not only the wind, but the weather in general, can raise your risk of a heart attack.

A study out of France found you're more likely to suffer a heart attack if the atmospheric pressure changes even 10 millibars, either up or down. What exactly does that mean? Meteorologist Dean Hutsell with the National Weather Service says this kind of change within a 24-hour period indicates a strong weather system — not necessarily a hurricane or a blizzard, but usually gusty winds, rain or snow, and a temperature change.

Whenever air masses move through an area, he says, there is a change in air pressure. The pressure falls as a system approaches, then rises after it passes. According to the study, these extreme changes raise your likelihood of having a first heart attack by about 11 percent. If you have suffered a previous heart attack, your risk is almost triple that.

The study found that cold weather may play a part as well. When temperatures fell 18 degrees below normal, heart attack risk rose 13 percent. The risk shot up to 38 percent in people who had suffered a previous heart attack. Past research has linked chilly temperatures to a rise in blood pressure, and researchers say that could be a factor.

So is there anything you can do to protect yourself from a weather-induced heart attack? Of course you can't change the weather, but you can take steps to minimize your risk.

▶ Pay attention to weather reports, especially if the forecast includes a drop in temperature or sudden change in atmospheric pressure.

▶ Insulate your house against drafts and the chill of winter.

▶ Dress warmly, both indoors and out.

► Stay cool and calm when a storm comes your way. Don't let thunder or lightning raise your stress level. Instead, take the opportunity to stay indoors and do something you find particularly restful and enjoyable.

Iron-clad heart protection

Want to help out your fellow man *and* reduce your risk of heart attack by an amazing 88 percent? Donate blood.

Researchers have found that too much iron in your system can nearly triple your heart attack risk. And by regularly donating blood, you are reducing your body's amount of stored iron.

Consider making an annual visit to the Red Cross if you:

• are a middle-aged male or a non-menstruating female.
• have had at least one heart attack.
• don't take antioxidant vitamins A, C, or E, or aspirin, which help counteract iron's oxidation process.

Heal your heart the Ornish way

It's a tough program, but if you can stick it out, you are almost guaranteed to reverse heart disease and lower your risk forever — without drugs or surgery. What is this revolutionary strategy? Dr. Dean Ornish's regimen of diet and lifestyle changes.

Ornish promises that by following his program you can improve your heart health even if you've been diagnosed with heart disease. In a recent trial, 82 percent of the participants experienced this kind of reversal just within the first year.

An early test of this program found that in only 24 days participants:

► reduced chest pain by 91 percent
► improved their ability to exercise
► reduced cholesterol levels by 21 percent
► felt less anxiety, fear, and depression

▶ had an improved sense of well-being

Ornish believes his lifestyle program is especially beneficial for people with slight hypertension (high blood pressure). In three research studies, he had to decrease or discontinue blood pressure medications for most of the participants. By changing their diet and lifestyle, the patients brought down their blood pressure naturally. The additional drugs were actually making their pressures too low and causing uncomfortable side effects.

To get similar results, here are the lifestyle changes you will have to make:

▶ eat a vegetarian diet of no more than 10 percent fat

▶ practice moderate daily aerobic exercise

▶ attend stress management training

▶ stop smoking

▶ attend group support meetings

Some critics say these changes are too drastic to be maintained for long. Others say they're not such a high price to pay for improved health. And studies show that your health will improve. Those following the Ornish plan in the most recent study, the five-year Lifestyle Heart Trial, suffered fewer heart attacks than those who made only moderate changes. They also needed less surgery, reversed their atherosclerosis, and reduced their LDL cholesterol levels.

Besides trimming your fat intake to just 10 percent of your total calories, Ornish also recommends eating lots of complex carbohydrates. They should make up the biggest chunk of your diet, he says, while only about 20 percent of your calories should come from protein. You should also try not to take in more than 5 milligrams of cholesterol a day.

All this may sound complicated, but you don't need to constantly count calories or fat grams. Just remember that the type of food you eat is more important than the amount.

Gather nature's harvest. Plant foods like fruits, vegetables, grains, and legumes are natural forms of complex carbohydrates. These are high in fiber and fill you up without adding lots of calories. By eating mostly plant foods, you'll be cutting fat and cholesterol.

Forget the fat. Avoid all oils and stay away from high-fat foods, even vegetarian ones like avocados, olives, coconut, nuts, seeds, and cocoa products.

Avoid animal products. With the exception of egg whites and one cup of nonfat yogurt or milk a day, for vitamin B12, you should avoid all animal products. No meat, poultry, seafood, or egg yolks.

Cut out caffeine. Try to avoid caffeine, which may worsen irregular heartbeats or provoke stress.

Say sayonara to sweets. Sugar, by itself, is not strongly linked to heart disease. It's just usually found in foods high in saturated fat and cholesterol. By avoiding one, you are avoiding the others.

Substitute for salt. Salt raises blood pressure in some people. If you are salt-sensitive, avoid it and add flavorings with other spices or vinegar. If not, use salt in moderation.

Adjust your alcohol. Limit alcohol to 2 ounces per day or less.

So what about all those other low-fat diets you've heard about? Most eating programs supported by the American Heart Association, the U.S. Department of Agriculture, and the U.S. Department of Health and Human Services recommend a total dietary fat intake of no more than 30 percent of your total calories. For example, if you are on a 2,000 calorie-a-day diet, they say you should eat no more than 600 fat calories a day. Ornish's program, on the other hand, allows only 200 fat calories a day.

Ornish claims these 30-percent-fat diets cannot improve heart health. You may slow down the progression of heart disease, he says, but it still gets worse.

Most experts do agree you must make sweeping changes in your total lifestyle. Just lowering the fat and cholesterol in your diet won't be enough to reduce your risk of heart disease, let alone improve your heart health. You need a combination of diet and lifestyle changes to see any improvements. That's where the exercise, no smoking, stress management, and support factors could make the difference.

To see the positive effects of this diet, Ornish recommends you follow his guidelines for at least three weeks. That's how long it takes to break bad habits and establish new, healthy ones.

Heartburn

20 ways to take the heat out of heartburn

If you suffer from burning pain, gas, belching, and bloating, you're not alone. More than half of adults get heartburn.

Also called acid indigestion or reflux, heartburn actually has nothing to do with your heart. It occurs when stomach acid flows back up your esophagus, the tube that carries food to your stomach. It can cause a burning pain behind your breastbone and into your neck and throat. Normally, a circular muscle, called a sphincter, separates your stomach and esophagus, keeping the acid where it belongs. But if this muscle becomes weak, it loses its ability to stay closed.

If heartburn pain is a frequent guest at your table, here are some things you can do to make your life more comfortable.

Eat less, more often. Small, frequent meals, say four to six light helpings a day, are healthier than three large ones. Avoid stuffing yourself.

Ban late-night snacks. Avoid eating just before bedtime. Don't even lie down for four hours after eating.

Think bland. Fatty and spicy dishes will irritate your stomach lining and esophagus. Some of the worst offenders are tomato products, onions, and peppers.

Choco-holics beware. Some experts claim that chocolate and chocolate drinks are the number one cause of heartburn. They'll have you doubled over before you can say "double fudge."

Say "no way" to oj. Stay away from citrus fruits and juices. A survey of 400 heartburn sufferers showed that grapefruit juice caused more heartburn than any other beverage, followed closely by orange juice and tomato-containing juices. These fruits are irritating because of their high acid content.

Pass on the after-dinner mint. Peppermint and spearmint may give you refreshing breath, but they can also give you heartburn.

Give your jaw a workout. The more you chew, the more acid-neutralizing saliva you produce. Take small bites and chew your food slowly and thoroughly. After eating, chew a piece of sugarless gum.

Watch what you drink. Cut down on coffee, tea, alcoholic beverages, and whole milk. These tend to irritate your stomach lining.

Timing is everything. Drink liquids about an hour before or after meals to keep your stomach from bloating. Don't mix foods and liquids.

Improve your posture. Sit up straight when you're eating — never stand or lie down. And don't bend over immediately after eating. This forces food and digestive acids back up into your esophagus.

Do one thing at a time. Don't eat while working, playing, or driving.

Avoid tight clothes. Don't wear clothes and belts that fit tightly around your stomach. Choose clothes that fit loosely at your waistline.

Slim down. If you are overweight, losing those extra pounds may help relieve your symptoms. The extra weight squeezes your belly and forces the acidic digestive juices back up into your windpipe.

Give up smoking. And if you're already trying to quit, don't wear your nicotine patch to bed. The nicotine it releases can cause heartburn.

Treat yourself. Suck on sugarless hard candy during the day, but avoid those that are peppermint flavored.

Get support while you sleep. Use 4- to 6-inch wooden blocks or bricks to raise the head of your bed. Or, put a foam wedge beneath your upper body. This keeps digestive juices flowing down instead of up as you sleep. Extra pillows usually won't do the trick. They merely force a bend at your waist.

Down the hatch. Drink plenty of water with your medications, and don't lie down after swallowing a pill. This helps the pills go down and stay down.

Take it easy. Avoid straining and heavy lifting. This causes your abdominal muscles to contract and squeeze the contents of your stomach up and into your esophagus.

Flush out your system. Drinking water throughout the day will help keep the digestive acids washed out of your esophagus.

Know your medications. Talk to your doctor if you are taking any heart or blood pressure medicines. These can affect the sphincter between your esophagus and stomach, allowing acid to back up into your esophagus.

If your heartburn ever becomes severe and is accompanied by nausea, sweating, weakness, fainting, or breathlessness, or pain that extends from your chest to your arm or jaw, you may have something much worse than a pepperoni pizza that didn't sit well. These symptoms could be indications of a heart attack. Call for emergency help.

When heartburn spells BIG trouble

Most people get heartburn now and then, and it's usually nothing to worry about. But if it comes back — again and again — it could be cause for concern.

Gastroesophageal reflux disease (GERD) is a general term for the symptoms of indigestion and acid reflux, also called heartburn. This condition occurs when acid from your stomach backs up into your esophagus, causing a burning sensation in your chest. If this happens often, the acid can damage your esophagus.

About one out of three adults has occasional heartburn, and out of these about 10 percent have it bad enough to develop Barrett's esophagus. This is a condition in which the body, in an effort to protect the esophagus from stomach acid, replaces the cells lining the esophagus with cells like those in the intestines. This increases your risk of cancer of the esophagus by as much as 40 times.

Most heartburn sufferers don't know heartburn can be dangerous. If you take an antacid for heartburn relief on more days than not, or your heartburn causes moderate pain, see your doctor. Catching the problem early can make a big difference in heading off Barrett's esophagus.

Perhaps most frightening of all is that the number of cases of GERD and Barrett's esophagus is rising. Some doctors point to obesity as a major cause of the recent increase. Obesity raises the pressure in your intestines and with it the risk of acid reflux. Simply put, if you've got too much in your gut, the excess has to go somewhere.

Diet may also play a role. The type of diet that can easily lead to obesity — too much fat and red meat and not enough fruits and vegetables — can also easily cause acid reflux.

The best thing you can do for your esophagus is to maintain a healthy weight. Follow your doctor's advice for quieting and preventing heartburn, and try some of the tips found in this chapter. With a few minor changes to your lifestyle, you should be able to avoid the discomfort of heartburn and keep your digestive system in good working order.

Don't get 'burned' on antacids

You've got heartburn. Pop a few antacids and you'll be as good as new. Right? Not if you suffer from the hidden side effects of many antacids.

Seltzer-type products contain a lot of salt and shouldn't be taken by people who are on low-sodium diets. Antacids that are high in calcium should be avoided by people with kidney problems. Calcium antacids can also cause a rebound effect, resulting in even greater acid production.

If your favorite heartburn remedy contains magnesium, don't take more than the recommended daily dose, and don't use it for more than a week without your doctor's approval. Otherwise, you could build up deadly levels of magnesium in your body. The elderly are especially vulnerable. Magnesium is excreted from your body by your kidneys, and kidney function decreases with age.

The signs of this dangerous side effect are low blood pressure, muscle weakness, lightheadedness, confusion, heart rhythm disturbances, nausea, and vomiting.

Besides checking your antacid for these ingredients, consider switching from the liquid type to the tablet form. Although many people think liquid antacids work better than tablet antacids, scientific evidence says otherwise.

Oklahoma researchers were surprised to find that tablets actually provide greater and longer-lasting relief than liquids. A study of 65 heartburn sufferers revealed that Tums E-X tablets and Mylanta Double Strength tablets controlled heartburn better than the liquid Mylanta II and Extra Strength Maalox.

The tablets did a better job of lowering acid levels in the esophagus and reducing the number of times stomach juices flowed back into the windpipe. In fact, two hours after taking the medicine, only people who had used the liquid antacids were still having heartburn.

The tablets mix with your saliva to form a gummy substance that sticks to your esophagus better and longer than the liquid medicine. Plus, the act of chewing the tablets may bring out the natural antacids in your saliva.

Delicious berry battles cancer

New research shows you might have another ally in the fight against cancer of the esophagus, and a delicious one at that — black raspberries.

In recent findings, test animals fed a diet containing 5 percent black raspberries developed 39 percent fewer tumors when injected with cancer-causing agents. When the amount of black raspberries was increased to 10 percent, there were 49 percent less tumors.

Doctors think an antioxidant in the berries, called ellagic acid, is mostly responsible for these remarkable results. Ellagic acid attacks damaging molecules that can lead to cancerous

growths. Another antioxidant present in black raspberries, vitamin C, might also lend a hand.

Other good sources of ellagic acid include strawberries,
grapefruit, and some nuts.

A mighty herb for a queasy stomach

When you think of chamomile, you probably think of one thing
— tea. But the truth is, chamomile not only makes great tea, it has
been used for centuries to treat a variety of ailments. The ancient
Egyptians used chamomile to treat everything from anxiety and
insomnia to dizziness, laryngitis, and skin conditions.

Today, this wonder herb is best known for relieving nausea, stomach cramps, and gas. Chamomile is also used as an additive in cosmetics and health products.

The high flavonoid content of chamomile makes it an important
cancer fighter. Some research suggests this remarkable little flower
helps to slow the growth of cancer cells. One of chamomile's active
ingredients is a powerful antioxidant that reduces inflammation.

Drinking chamomile tea is the most popular way to enjoy its benefits. The recommended dose is a cup of water brewed with two or
three teaspoons of dried or fresh flower heads, steeped for 10 minutes. This can be taken up to three times a day.

With more and more health experts getting wise to the benefits
of herbal medicine, chamomile might soon prove to be the cure-all
of the century.

Hemorrhoids

8 things you can do to find relief

Even though half of adults over 50 have hemorrhoids, that doesn't mean you should ignore them.

These swollen veins can occur inside the rectum or bulge outside the anus. Both kinds can become itchy and painful, and they can also bleed.

There's no reason to live with the pain. Give these natural remedies a try, but if your condition worsens or doesn't improve within seven days, or if bleeding occurs, see your doctor.

Fight back with fiber. The number one way to prevent and treat hemorrhoids is to add fiber to your diet. Fiber will help you avoid constipation, soften your stool, and relieve the pressure on your hemorrhoids.

Try to get about 25 to 30 grams of fiber each day. Good sources are bran, whole grain foods, potatoes, beans, and fresh fruits. To really get things moving, eat more vegetables like cabbage, corn, parsnips, brussels sprouts, cauliflower, peas, asparagus, carrots, and kale.

Foods low in fiber will only slow up the process and make your stools harder to pass. Avoid ice cream, soft drinks, cheese, white bread, and meat. In addition, some people find that certain foods, like coffee, nuts, or spicy foods, make their hemorrhoid symptoms worse.

Take it "sitting" down. If your hemorrhoids are inflamed, soaking in a few inches of warm water with your knees raised will really ease your pain. Try three 15-minute soaks a day to soothe your uncomfortable symptoms. Don't make the water too hot, and don't add anything like bubble bath or Epsom salts — these can irritate swollen veins. You can relax in your tub or find Sitz Baths at your local pharmacy, very reasonably priced.

Practice proper bathroom etiquette. Straining during a bowel movement is one of the major causes of hemorrhoids. To prevent this, take a footstool into the bathroom and prop up your feet. If you don't have a stool, anything that raises your feet at least a few inches will do.

Try gently lubricating the area, inside and out, with nonpetroleum jelly first. You may find bowel movements less irritating.

And although you shouldn't rush the process, don't sit too long either. Enjoying your favorite magazine for more than a few minutes increases the pressure on the veins in your rectum. The longer you sit, the more your veins swell.

Last, but not least, clean well. If the area is particularly sensitive after a bowel movement, wipe with a soft, moist tissue or baby wipes instead of regular toilet tissue.

Flush it out. Six to eight glasses of liquid each day will flush out your digestive system and keep it from becoming impacted. Stay away from alcohol because it draws water from your body and causes constipation.

Stay active. Hemorrhoids should not restrict your normal exercise routine. In fact, it's more important than ever for you to exercise every day — for two reasons. First of all, moving around instead of sitting takes pressure off the veins in your rectum. And secondly, exercise helps prevent constipation, one of the main causes of hemorrhoids. Just avoid heavy lifting and any activity that causes you to strain.

Slim down. Being overweight is often a consequence of an inactive lifestyle and poor diet. Changing these two aspects of your life will improve your health, including the condition of your hemorrhoids.

Cool the heat. If your hemorrhoids are painfully swollen, take this as an excuse to rest. Stay in bed for a few hours with an ice pack on your anal area.

Reach for over-the-counter help. There are several products you can buy for different kinds of hemorrhoid relief. Bulk stool softeners are helpful, but stay away from laxatives. Diarrhea is just as bad for hemorrhoids as constipation. External creams or ointments for pain, swelling, and itching usually contain a lubricant to relieve irritation, but nonpetroleum jelly does the same job. If you choose a commercial product, these are some helpful ingredients:

▶ Hydrocortisone — relieves inflammation and itching.

▶ Anesthetics (benzocaine, pramoxine) — can numb the pain.

▶ Vasoconstrictors (ephedrine, phenylephrine) — reduce swelling and relieve itching.

▶ Astringents (witch hazel, zinc oxide) — help shrink blood vessels.

▶ Counterirritants (camphor) — soothe and comfort the area.

▶ Aloe vera gel — reduces irritation.

Particular brands may list other ingredients, such as wound-healing agents and antiseptics, but not all of these have been proven useful.

Explosive new treatment for hemorrhoids

Need guaranteed pain relief from your hemorrhoids? Talk to your doctor about nitroglycerin ointment. This cream contains a low dose of nitroglycerin, about the same amount used in tablets to prevent angina attacks. But now researchers have found that it dramatically relieves the pain of hemorrhoids and ulcers on the anus, called anal fissures.

Since the Food and Drug Administration (FDA) has not yet approved nitroglycerin ointment for this kind of treatment, you can only get it through your doctor.

Overcome pain with herbal remedies

If you like using natural treatments, try one of these herbs for hemorrhoid relief.

Butcher's broom. This herb reduces inflammation and shrinks veins.

Witch hazel. Forms a protective layer over your skin, which allows it to heal. This is important in preventing hemorrhoids from recurring. It also relieves itching and inflammation.

Myrrh. It's an antiseptic that can be used on external hemorrhoids.

Plantain or psyllium seeds. They are used as a bulk laxative. This means if you take them with lots of water, they swell up and move through your digestive system quickly. This process softens your stool, reduces the straining of constipation, and relieves bleeding and pain during bowel movements.

Hiccups

17 hiccup remedies that really work

Man can walk on the moon and create computers the size of a fingernail, but hiccups remain a mystery. Unfortunately, curing them is just as puzzling. Although doctors have tried everything from drugs to hypnosis, these old-fashioned home remedies work just as well.

Change the pressure in your sinuses. By plugging up your ear canal, you are increasing the pressure inside your sinuses. This could force the muscle spasm that caused the hiccup to relax.

- ▶ plug up one ear with your finger
- ▶ plug both ears and drink a glass of water

Master some massage therapy. Many experts believe the part of your body that controls hiccups is in the upper part of your spinal column, in the back of your neck. Several of these remedies apply pressure to nerve centers that may be connected to this control site.

- ▶ pull gently on your tongue
- ▶ massage your earlobes
- ▶ with a spoon, lift the uvula (the small tissue hanging down at the back of your throat)
- ▶ pinch your upper lip, just below your right nostril
- ▶ apply gentle pressure to your closed eyelids

Stimulate your throat. The nerves at the back of your throat may trigger the muscle spasm causing your hiccups. By distracting those nerves with something else, you may be able to stop the hiccups.

- ▶ sip ice water
- ▶ gargle

▶ swallow some sugar

▶ bite on a lemon

▶ drink from the far side of a glass of water

Check your breathing. The idea is to interrupt the hiccup cycle by stopping the flow of oxygen for a short time.

▶ draw your knees to your chest and wrap your arms around them and squeeze

▶ hold your breath

▶ sneeze

▶ cough

▶ breathe into a paper bag

High Blood Pressure

3 minerals attack silent killer

High blood pressure is called the silent killer because it doesn't have any symptoms. Many people don't even know they have it. Left untreated, it can lead to heart attack, stroke, congestive heart failure, kidney damage, and atherosclerosis.

To make your high blood pressure do a disappearing act, be sure you're getting enough of these three "magic" minerals.

► **Calcium.** This bone-building mineral keeps your muscles, including your heart, strong and working efficiently. It also works to keep your blood pressure normal. Good sources of calcium are low-fat milk and yogurt, cooked turnip greens, canned salmon, and cottage cheese. The best way to eat calcium-rich foods is in small meals and simple combinations, like cereal with milk. You can also buy calcium supplements. To absorb the calcium you need, you must have a sufficient amount of vitamin D in your body. Vitamin D is added to most milk, but you can also get it by spending some time outside. Your body produces vitamin D when it's exposed to the sun. Check with your doctor before deciding how much calcium to take.

► **Magnesium.** A new study shows this mineral can lower blood pressure. In the study, 60 people with high blood pressure were treated with a magnesium supplement or a fake pill. After eight weeks, the people taking the magnesium supplements had a significant drop in blood pressure. The higher the blood pressure, the more it decreased. To get magnesium naturally, eat fresh and unprocessed foods. Avocados, raw sunflower seeds and almonds, pinto beans, black-eyed peas, spinach, baked potatoes, and broccoli are good sources.

▶ **Potassium.** When it comes to lowering blood pressure, potassium packs a powerful punch. Scientists began studying the effects of potassium on high blood pressure as early as 1928. Now a major study of 300 nurses shows that potassium can lower your blood pressure even if it's in the normal range. Good sources of potassium are dried apricots, avocados, dried figs, acorn squash, baked potatoes, kidney beans, cantaloupe, citrus fruits, and bananas. You can also buy potassium supplements. If you're taking a diuretic, your body is getting rid of potassium along with fluid. Ask your doctor if you are taking a potassium-sparing diuretic. If not, make sure you eat more potassium-rich foods. If you have any kidney damage, check with your doctor before increasing your potassium intake.

Put the brakes on blood pressure naturally

High blood pressure puts you at risk for a number of health problems. That's why keeping your blood pressure in check is an important goal. Here are some simple but effective strategies:

- **Keep your weight down.** For people who are overweight, losing weight is one of the most effective ways to lower blood pressure.
- **Eat less fat.** Too much dietary fat and cholesterol can clog arteries damaged by high blood pressure and cause atherosclerosis.
- **Watch your salt intake.** If you are salt-sensitive, eating less salt can help lower your blood pressure.
- **Exercise regularly.** This is good for your overall health, but it also helps lower blood pressure.
- **Stop smoking.** A person who smokes and has high blood pressure is three to five times more likely to die from heart disease than a nonsmoker.
- **Limit alcohol.** Even without other risk factors, drinking too much alcohol can cause high blood pressure. Don't drink more than 2 ounces of liquor, 8 ounces of wine, or 24 ounces of beer a day.

Beware of the 'grapefruit effect'

Grapefruit juice in the morning may be nutritious and delicious, but it could cause your blood pressure drug to build up to toxic levels in your body.

The "grapefruit effect" on drugs was discovered accidentally by researchers several years ago when they gave volunteers grapefruit juice to hide the taste of a medication. They found out that when the medicine was taken with grapefruit juice, it multiplied the amount of the medication in the blood.

Later studies found that grapefruit contains a substance called DHB that blocks the effects of an enzyme, which helps break down certain types of drugs in your body. Instead of being metabolized, the drugs continue to circulate in your body and accumulate.

The "grapefruit effect" has been beneficial to some people, including transplant recipients. Although the grapefruit effect could help make some drugs more effective, consider the American Heart Association's recommendation — don't drink grapefruit juice about the same time as taking calcium channel blockers.

The same thing happens with Seville oranges because, like grapefruit, they contain DHB. But since you're likely to eat Seville oranges only in marmalade — and a spoonful of marmalade probably doesn't contain enough DHB to affect your medication — the risk is small.

Other drugs that may be affected by grapefruit juice include some types of sleeping pills, antihistamines, and cyclosporine. Ask your doctor or pharmacist if grapefruit juice will affect your medication.

Gourmet coffee just got better

If your idea of great coffee is a steaming cup of espresso, but you worry about the caffeine — relax. The latest research proves espresso isn't as bad as you think.

As a matter of fact, a gleaming little 2-ounce cup contains less caffeine than a regular cup of drip or brewed coffee. Drip or brewed coffees can have 80 to 175 milligrams (mg) of caffeine per cup, while 1.5 to 2 ounces of espresso contain only 60 to 120 mg of caffeine. If the espresso is made with Arabica beans instead of Robusta beans, you'll get even less caffeine.

Why isn't gourmet coffee as caffeine-powered as you thought? First, espresso machines are fast. The ground beans don't stay in steaming water very long, so less caffeine seeps out than in a drip or brewed coffee maker. Second, the serving size is smaller than regular coffee.

Add milk to your dark-brewed espresso, and you'll offset a possible long-term side effect of caffeine — an increase in your need for calcium.

What about popular cappuccinos and lattes? Just be aware that a double latte contains two servings of espresso. Otherwise, these specialty coffees are not a big problem from a caffeine standpoint. Go easy on the sugar and take yours with skim or low-fat milk, and you can enjoy your morning pick-me-up or after-dinner java with peace of mind and no jitters.

Great-tasting salt substitute lowers blood pressure

About 60 percent of people who have high blood pressure are sensitive to salt. That means the more salt you eat, the higher your blood pressure goes. If you're a salt-sensitive person, most doctors recommend that you cut your daily salt consumption to 2,000 milligrams (mg) a day, which translates to about a teaspoon of salt.

Most of the salt in your diet is hidden in processed foods and fast foods. You can cut out a lot of salt simply by making healthier choices.

Lemon juice, herbs, and balsamic vinegar are tasty salt substitutes. You can also lessen your desire for salty foods by simply cutting out salt for a while. But if there are some foods you simply can't stomach without a little sprinkle of salt, you're in luck.

A reduced-sodium table "salt" may be the answer. Available at pharmacies and by mail order on the Internet, Cardia Salt contains less than half the sodium of regular salt. It also has added potassium and magnesium, two minerals that people with high blood pressure need more of. Several medical studies have shown that using Cardia

Salt for cooking and seasoning at the table can lower both systolic and diastolic blood pressure. According to the people in the study, there's one thing that makes this salt substitute stand out from the others — it tastes just like the real thing.

Dr. Paul K. Whelton, Dean of the School of Public Health at Tulane University, is one of the doctors who conducted a study of Cardia Salt. According to Dr. Whelton, "Many people are just above the threshold of being classified as hypertensive {having high blood pressure}." For those people, he believes, a product such as Cardia Salt might make enough difference to control blood pressure.

Dr. Whelton and his colleagues estimate that "A 2-mm Hg reduction in the average level of blood pressure in the entire population should result in a 17-percent reduction in the occurrence of hypertension, a 14-percent reduction in the average annual incidence of stroke, and a 6-percent reduction in the average annual incidence of coronary heart disease." Those are big improvements for such a small change.

If you are salt-sensitive and have high blood pressure, eating less salt is a small step that could pay big dividends. Ask your doctor about Cardia Salt. It might help get your blood pressure going in the right direction.

Natural treatment outshines the rest

Sunlight is vital to maintaining normal blood pressure. That's because vitamin D, the sunshine vitamin, helps your body absorb calcium, which regulates blood pressure.

That's the premise scientists were investigating in a recent study of 18 people with high blood pressure. For six weeks, the study participants were exposed to either ultraviolet B light or ultraviolet A light all over their bodies for short periods of time.

The people exposed to ultraviolet B light had a significant reduction in blood pressure. This is the same kind of light therapy people with psoriasis sometimes undergo, and the effect is similar to exposure to sunlight. The researchers think this reduction was caused by the connection between calcium and vitamin D.

Researchers also believe light directly affects blood pressure. Studies have shown that blood pressure tends to rise the farther you are from the equator and is higher in winter than in summer. It also tends to occur more often in dark-skinned people, who have more pigment in their skin to resist sunlight. Since the production of vitamin D in your body depends on the amount of sunlight you are exposed to, this could explain such differences in blood pressure.

If you want a natural prescription for lowering your high blood pressure, try a little dose of sunshine. You don't want to overdo it and get a sunburn, but a half-hour daily walk in the sunlight is good for two reasons. You'll be getting regular exercise, a good tonic for high blood pressure, and you'll be getting a dose of vitamin D.

Beware of sodium in your water

Many people don't like "hard" water. It's loaded with minerals, which is why it stains fixtures and doesn't lather well. If you think the solution is a water softening system — think again. This process removes the heart friendly minerals calcium and magnesium and adds sodium to the water.

A recent study found that the amount of sodium in some softened water may be enough to affect the blood pressure of salt-sensitive people.

The Michigan study tested samples from 59 homes with softened well water. The average concentration of sodium in the water was 278 milligrams (mg) per liter (about a quart). The sodium level of the water in 10 of the homes was more than 400 mg per liter. Keep in mind the recommended daily intake of sodium is 2,400 mg or less.

Some new water softening systems use potassium instead of sodium to soften water. If you are sensitive to salt but have no problems handling extra potassium, one of these systems might be a better choice for you.

Impotence

Foods that feed your sex life

Your diet can have a major impact on your sexual health. Since more than eight out of 10 cases of impotence can be traced to physical causes, taking care of yourself physically is one of the best ways to prevent it from happening to you. It all starts with what you put in your mouth and what you leave on the table.

Forego the fat. High-fat foods in particular can really foul up your sex life. Too much saturated fat and cholesterol in your diet can lead to high blood pressure and heart disease, and can make it harder for your blood vessels to get blood to where it needs to be during sex. In fact, a high total cholesterol count doubles a man's risk of becoming impotent.

In one study, doctors watched for impotence in 3,250 men, ages 25 through 83. Those men whose cholesterol was higher than 240 mg/dl were twice as likely to have a bout with impotence as those whose levels were below 180 mg/dl. Having too little HDL (good) cholesterol produced the same result, raising the risk of impotence just as much. So you need to watch your intake, and limit yourself to no more than 300 mg of cholesterol per day.

And if all that's not enough to send you to the salad bar once in a while, think about this — many of the common medications prescribed for high blood pressure today are known to cause impotence themselves. So don't count on your heart pills to save your sex life.

Eat "sex-friendly" foods. The best foods you can eat to protect your sexual health are those that make up a well-balanced, healthy diet. A healthy body that feels good is much more prepared for a good sex life than one whose nutritional balance is out of whack. And while they still haven't invented the sandwich that will turn you into Romeo, there are some "sex-friendly" foods you shouldn't overlook.

▶ **Fruits and veggies.** The antioxidants in most fruits and vegetables protect your cells from the attack of free radicals. Vitamins A, C, and E are perhaps the strongest at stopping free radicals from damaging your body, including the parts that need to be in tip-top shape for sex. As you know by now, fruits and vegetables might be the only thing you can't eat too much of, so point your cart in the direction of the produce aisle.

▶ **Fiber.** One of the ways fiber helps you sexually is by binding up cholesterol and removing it from your system. At least 30 grams of fiber from grains, cereals, fruits, and vegetables every day can help keep cholesterol out of your arteries, and high blood pressure (and frustration) out of your sex life.

▶ **Garlic.** You might think that something as strong smelling as garlic would hurt your love life more than it would help, but that's not the case. Some studies have shown that eating just half a clove per day can bring your cholesterol down about 9 percent. It can also help lower your blood pressure, and better blood flow means better sex. Garlic is also available in supplement form in case you're still concerned about your breath.

▶ **Oysters.** It sounds like a cliché, an old wives' tale. But the reason oysters have long been considered an aphrodisiac might be because of their high zinc content. Zinc is critical for the production of sperm, semen and testosterone, so adding more zinc to your diet could well add more spice to your love life. Other good sources of zinc include red meat and green, leafy spinach.

Following a sensible diet can help prevent impotence in your future. If you already have a problem, don't be embarrassed to see your doctor. Successful treatment is possible in 95 percent of the cases, yet only 5 percent of men seek help. A combination of treatments, including the right foods, may be just what you need to get your love life back on track.

Pelvic exercises may cure impotence

Just as you have muscles that allow you to walk, talk, and breathe, you have muscles that affect your ability to achieve and maintain an erection. In many cases, getting these muscles back into shape can eliminate impotence once and for all.

Pelvic muscle exercises, called Kegels, are designed to help you do just that. Women have been practicing them for years to help firm vaginal muscles, particularly after childbirth. Now researchers have found that these exercises help men as well.

In one study, a team of Belgian urologists treated 150 men who suffered from impotence. Some men had operations, and others did Kegel exercises. One year after treatment, 58 percent of the men who performed the Kegels were completely cured or were so satisfied with their improvement that they did not opt for surgery.

This routine developed by therapists at Boston's Beth Israel Hospital may be just what you need to regain control of your sex life.

▶ Squeeze your pelvic muscles as if you're trying to stop a flow of urine. You should feel your anal pelvic muscles contract also. Hold for 10 seconds, then relax for 10 seconds.

▶ Repeat this cycle up to 15 times, or until you can no longer hold the flex for a full 10 seconds.

▶ Take a few minutes to relax.

▶ Now do a fast set. Squeeze for a second and relax for a second, 10 times in a row.

▶ Do 10 sets of these, resting between sets.

You can perform these exercises as often as you like or as often as your doctor says you can. Be patient and stick to the program, and you should begin to see benefits before long.

Kegels can also be used to combat another frustrating problem — incontinence. Follow the same steps listed above, but add this extra technique.

▶ When urinating, use your pelvic muscles to stop the flow of urine in mid-stream. Repeat several times until your bladder is empty.

If you do this every time you urinate, the extra practice will help strengthen your muscles and control. During situations that cause leakage, constrict your pelvic muscles just as you do when practicing Kegels. Pretty soon, you'll be able to prevent most accidents just by squeezing your new, stronger muscles.

'Bark' up the right herbal tree

Since Viagra was approved, hundreds of thousands of men have flocked to the drug store for the little blue pills. Others, worried about reports over Viagra-related deaths, have stayed away. These men, and perhaps you as well, might prefer an herbal solution that has been around for more than 70 years. It's called yohimbine, but beware — it has a similar-sounding cousin that could be deadly if taken by mistake.

Yohimbine is a prescription-only impotence treatment made from the bark of an African tree. Before Viagra, it was the only impotence medication approved by the Food and Drug Administration. Although its effectiveness in humans has never been conclusively proven, some studies have shown it to have positive effects on erectile dysfunction, consistently performing better than a placebo in tests.

You may see a similar herbal solution, called yohimbe, in your local herb store. It's made from the same tree bark as yohimbine but is much more dangerous. Reactions to yohimbe have included high blood pressure, irregular heartbeat, vomiting, even paralysis and death if overdosed.

Although prescription yohimbine is not as dangerous as its cousin yohimbe, it does cause side effects in some people, including nausea, dizziness, nervousness, and headaches.

So if herbal's the way you prefer to deal with impotence, use caution. Prescription yohimbine might be just the thing for you. But watch out for over-the-counter remedies that may give you more than you ask for.

Insomnia

Sleep soundly without dangerous drugs

No matter what your age, a good night's sleep restores your body and clears your mind. But if you're older, you may find it particularly difficult to fall asleep at night or get back to sleep if you wake up early. Experts estimate that up to a quarter of all healthy seniors suffer from chronic insomnia.

Sleeping pills may seem like the only solution when you've spent countless nights tossing and turning. But the worst thing you can do is turn to drugs to relieve your sleeplessness. Although they may be necessary in some cases, they often do more harm than good.

Don't sabotage your sleep with drugs. Sleeping pills are a short-term solution for insomnia because the drugs lose their effectiveness after a few weeks. And in the meantime, they can cause a number of distressing side effects, such as daytime drowsiness, a hangover feeling, or nightmares.

Sleep medications may interfere with your normal sleep patterns and can, in fact, cause rebound insomnia. This means after you quit taking them, your sleep problem gets worse.

Fortunately, scientists have proven there is a better way to get enough sleep. In a research study of healthy seniors with insomnia, they compared sleeping pills and Cognitive-Behavior Training (CBT), a program of education and habit changes.

In the early part of the study, sleeping improved for all participants except those taking a placebo, a sleeping pill with no active ingredients. But follow-ups one and two years later showed that only the CBT group continued to sleep significantly better.

Cognitive-behavior therapy can teach you new ways to think about sleep and help you break the unhealthy patterns you've developed. Here are some ways you can put your sleep problems to rest permanently.

Look at sleep with a new attitude. You've heard you should sleep at least eight hours a night, so you worry when you don't measure up. Or you think the more time you spend in bed, the more rest you'll get, so you toss and turn trying to force yourself to sleep. Mistaken beliefs like these could be what's keeping you from a peaceful night's rest.

▶ Not everybody requires eight hours of sleep. How well you sleep is more important than how much time you spend in slumber.

▶ Spending a lot of time in bed doesn't help you sleep more.

▶ Sleeping patterns change with age. Nighttime sleep is more often interrupted with periods of wakefulness, and less time is spent in deep sleep. But if you feel alert and energetic during the day, you probably are getting plenty of good sleep.

▶ Everything that goes wrong on a bad day isn't necessarily related to sleep loss. Look for other causes and what you can do to change things.

Change your sleep pattern. Try limiting your time in bed to just the amount of time you are already sleeping. This will train your body to sleep and wake on a regular schedule.

▶ If you think you sleep about six hours a night, even though you are in bed eight hours, start spending no more than six hours in bed. Allow at least five hours, even if you think you sleep less.

▶ When you regularly sleep most of the six hours, add 15 to 20 minutes more to your time in bed, gradually increasing the length of your night's sleep.

Learn new bedtime habits. You need to associate the bedroom and bedtime with sleeping, not worrying about sleeping. Make these changes in your habits and see if your sleep improves.

▶ Wait until you are really sleepy to go to bed.

► Just use the bedroom for sleeping and sex. No reading, watching TV, or any other activity — including worrying — day or night. Anything that stimulates alertness should be done in another place.

► If you don't fall asleep within 15 to 20 minutes, get out of bed and go into a different room until sleepy again. Repeat this as often as necessary when trying to fall asleep. Don't "try harder." Sleep cannot be forced.

► Get up at the same time every morning, no matter how much — or how little— you have slept.

► Catnaps during the day are OK for older folks. But limit them to an hour, and don't nap after 3:00 p.m.

For a little more help, you might try a warm drink, a back rub, or a relaxation tape. In a hospital experiment, researchers found that older people reduced their use of sleeping pills substantially when they used these pleasant alternatives.

10 natural ways to end sleepless nights

Some people spend each night in peaceful slumber. They wake up refreshed, with energy to spare. If you, on the other hand, find yourself dragging sleepily through another day, don't despair. These tips will help you end your restless nights and feel more rejuvenated each day.

Keep a regular sleep schedule. Wait until you are really sleepy to go to bed. But have a regular time to settle down for the night. This way you will establish a rhythm to help trigger sleep. And get up at the same time every morning even if you didn't sleep well the night before. Stick to this schedule on weekends as well.

Enjoy a relaxing routine before bedtime. Take a warm bath, and add a touch of lavender scent if you find it soothing. Lower the lights, and listen to some soft music. Don't watch stimulating television shows or read upsetting news stories. And wait until morning when you are fresh and rested to write those checks to pay your bills.

Make your bedroom an inviting place for sleep. Be sure you have a comfortable bed and pillow. Keep your room dark — perhaps with window shades or heavy drapes. To shut out bothersome sounds, you may want to purchase a white noise machine or wear ear plugs. Most people say they sleep better in a cool room, but keep it at whatever temperature is comfortable for you.

Exercise, but not within a few hours before bedtime. Slumber usually comes easier to people who get regular exercise. Some sleep research seems to show that afternoon is the best time. But make it early. If you exercise too close to bedtime, it can be stimulating rather than relaxing.

Limit caffeine, alcohol, and nicotine. Have no more than two cups of coffee a day, none after noon. And limit tea, colas, and chocolate as well. They also contain caffeine.

Alcohol may make falling asleep easier, but wakefulness will follow. So don't drink any in the evening if you truly want to sleep tight. And nicotine is a stimulant, so don't smoke before bedtime or during the night.

Avoid a big meal before bedtime. A busy digestive system can really interfere with peaceful sleep. You should especially stay away from spicy foods late in the day.

But a glass of warm milk may be just the nightcap you need. You'll get calcium and magnesium, two minerals that are important in producing melatonin, which controls your sleep cycle.

Have a cup of valerian tea. For a relaxing brew, add two teaspoons of dried valerian root to a cup of hot water. It seems to work best for insomnia in older folks. There don't seem to be any side effects with occasional use.

Don't look at your clock during the night. It may be better not to know how long you have been tossing and turning. You are likely to stay awake even longer worrying about it. And if the ticking or luminous dial bothers you, remove it from the bedroom.

Spend some time outdoors in the morning sun. You can sleep better at night if you soak up some bright light early in the day.

Morning sunshine increases the level of melatonin in your body. This hormone helps regulate your sleep cycle naturally.

Practice gradual relaxation. If you are too tense to sleep, try relaxing your muscles, one group at a time. Beginning with your toes, work your way up — feet, calves, thighs, abdomen, hips, and so forth — until you reach your scalp. By that point, you should be relaxed and ready for sleep.

If you want to be at your best during the day, make sure you get enough quality shut-eye every night. With these new sleep-time habits, you'll soon be off to pleasant dreams.

Taming the wide-awake vacation blues

You've dreamed of a summer vacation in the Rocky Mountains, and suddenly here you are. Now all you need is a good night's sleep, and you'll be ready to jump right into your new adventures. But it's past midnight, and you are wide awake.

Adjust to the altitude. It's not just your excitement. Sleep disturbances are common at high altitudes — at least at first. It may be due to the thinner oxygen, which causes changes in your breathing. The higher up you go, the more likely you are to be affected.

You may want to rethink your plans and start out a little slower. Cutting your activities to just a half day on the first few days will help your body adjust to the new altitude. Most people adapt completely to new altitudes within two or three weeks.

Zone in on a new sleep cycle. If you have come from a different time zone, it's possible you are suffering from jet lag. This happens because your body is still on a sleep cycle that is out of sync with the sun in the new location.

It may help to have your meals, go to bed, and get up according to the new time right away. And get outside during the day. Sunlight will help your biological clock change faster, while staying indoors will only make your jet lag worse.

Prepare for the unfamiliar. To make your first nights away from home less stressful, try these comfort boosters.

▶ Take along a few favorite objects — like your pillow or some family photographs. They'll make your new surroundings seem more familiar.

▶ Before turning in for the night, tighten your draperies against outside light.

▶ Turn on the radio between stations for static "white noise" to block out unfamiliar sounds.

With a few adjustments — plus a little time — sleep disturbances won't interfere with your vacation fun.

Irritable Bowel Syndrome

New relief for irritable bowel syndrome

For many years, doctors recommended eating bran to get rid of the painful symptoms of irritable bowel syndrome (IBS) and to ease digestion. But research suggests that bran may not be the best remedy for your problem. In fact, some findings indicate it is five times more likely to hurt than to help.

IBS is a difficult condition to diagnose because experts don't know what causes it, and many of its symptoms mimic other conditions. One person might suffer from mild bloating and gas, while another experiences severe cramping, diarrhea, or constipation. But if you're like most people, you've probably followed the advice of doctors and nutritionists who told you to include plenty of bran and other high-fiber grains in your diet. And you may have ended up with a more irritated bowel than ever.

Choose the right foods. Instead of bran and other grains, try getting your fiber from gentler sources such as fruits and cooked vegetables. Researchers have found that these produce better results with far less chance of abdominal pain and bowel disturbance. Psyllium, the dried seed husks of a certain type of plantain, is another natural way to help regulate yourself. It can be found in such over-the-counter products as Metamucil.

Try the "exclusion" diet. If eating fiber seems to do more harm than good, try this special diet that relieved symptoms for IBS sufferers in a British study. Researchers found that symptoms improved for subjects whose diet excluded beef, dairy products, and all cereals except rice. You also need to cut back on yeast, citrus fruits, caffeinated drinks, and tap water. Try it for two weeks, and see how your body responds.

The British researchers think certain high-fiber foods may cause extra fermentation in the bowels, which leads to more gas and intestinal discomfort. Fermentation also may produce other chemicals that affect your bowels or nervous system. By restricting your diet, you should produce less gas, which may help relieve your symptoms.

Manage your stress. By reducing stress in your life, you may give your digestive system a break. Your system is very sensitive to stress, and many feel that stress and activities that tax your body in general are particularly harsh on your bowels. Try exercise or meditation to help manage your IBS symptoms.

Keep a journal. Although most doctors do not believe food allergies cause IBS, it is known that food sensitivities do. A good way to determine what foods may cause flare-ups is to keep an IBS journal. When you experience symptoms, record what you have eaten recently as well as your activities and any stress you may be under. By keeping such a journal, you may see patterns forming and can prevent further outbreaks by avoiding their causes.

Top herbal healers for IBS pain

If changing your eating habits doesn't relieve your discomfort, it's time for alternative measures. Try these herbs to see if they help calm some of your painful symptoms.

Peppermint oil. It may not sound like a soothing solution, but many people with IBS swear by it. In a recent hospital test, patients who took peppermint oil capsules 15 to 30 minutes before meals had about an 80 percent reduction in symptoms, including abdominal pain and distention, stomach growling, and flatulence.

By swallowing a special enteric-coated capsule, you can be sure it dissolves in your intestines where it will do the most good, and not in your stomach where it could irritate you even more. Try taking one or two 0.2 milliliter (ml) capsules three times a day between meals.

Chamomile. This herb has been shown to offer soothing relief from IBS symptoms. To relieve cramps and intestinal irritation, you can steep the dried flowers and drink it as a tea, or mix an alcohol-based tincture of chamomile with hot water. Some herbal experts recommend drinking either brew three or four times a day between meals.

Flaxseed. This seed has been used for centuries as a laxative. Its high-fiber content is a plus for your whole digestive system. To help with the constipation, gas, and inflamed colon of IBS, mix one tablespoon of whole or bruised flaxseed into 150 ml of liquid, and drink two or three times a day. You can sprinkle whole flaxseed on cereal or a salad to add a nutty, healthy flair.

Leg Pain

Get a leg up on leg pain

One of the most painful and frustrating interruptions to a good night's rest or an afternoon stroll is a sudden cramp. Unfortunately, leg cramps are extremely common and can be caused by problems in your diet, your exercise routine, or your sleeping patterns. The good news is, most leg pain is easily treated, and in fact, even more easily prevented.

Drink lots of fluids. Dehydration is probably the number one source of cramps. When your body loses too much water, it has a tendency to let you know, and cramping is one way it does this. To keep one step ahead of cramps, make sure you drink at least eight glasses of water every day.

Watch your mineral count. A proper diet is a great safeguard against cramping and other forms of leg pain, and several key minerals will form your first line of defense. If leg pain is a problem for you, paying special attention to these minerals will make sure that cramps don't have a chance to creep up on you.

► **Potassium.** You probably know that bananas are a good source of potassium. But if you really want your fill of this important mineral, try a cup of dried apricots or figs, or a rich, ripe avocado. They each have more than 1,000 milligrams. Potassium also is widely available in supplement form, as are the other important anti-cramp minerals.

► **Magnesium.** Keep up your magnesium stores with a few almonds or cashews, apricots, whole grains, soybeans, or dark-green leafy vegetables.

▶ **Calcium.** What's good for the bone is good for the muscle, so drink your milk. Yogurt and other forms of dairy work too, of course, as well as dried peas and beans, and dark-green leafy vegetables.

Try a tonic. High doses of quinine may cut down on nighttime leg cramps but can also lead to a scary parade of side effects. That's why the FDA has banned over-the-counter and prescription quinine pills for leg cramps. But you might find some relief if you drink a cup of tonic water before you go to bed. An 8-ounce glass contains 27 milligrams of quinine, which is enough to tame muscle cramps in some people. If you find it too bitter, mix the tonic water with lemon or orange juice.

What if a cramp slips through your defenses? Don't panic. Follow these easy steps to rid your muscle of its uninvited guest:

▶ **Keep it down.** As soon as you feel a cramp coming on, lower that part of your body to a level beneath the rest of your body. This keeps blood circulating more freely to the cramped area. If the cramp comes at night, just hang your arm or leg over the side of your bed.

▶ **Turn up the heat.** Adding some heat to the situation can help ease your pain. Blankets, hot baths, and heating pads can all do the trick, but take care — too much heat can actually enlarge your blood vessels, causing other circulation problems down the road.

▶ **Get your flex time.** When the cramp hits, don't grab and rub. Instead, sit and flex. There will be time enough later to rub your sore muscle, but right now, the best thing for it is to stop the spasm. Sit up in bed, straighten your leg, grab the ball of your foot, and stretch it toward you. Hold your leg in this position until the cramp relaxes. Practicing this flex move every day — with or without a cramp — will help keep your leg muscles in shape and lower your chances of suffering a painful charlie horse.

No-sweat defense against cramps

They say an ounce of prevention is worth a pound of cure. That may or may not be true, but in the case of cramps, a little preparation is better than waking up at 2:00 a.m. with your legs on fire. Use this special stretching technique to keep your calf muscles limber and pain-free.

With your shoes off, stand about two to three feet away from a wall. Placing your hands flat on the wall, lean forward, being careful to keep your back and legs straight and your heels pressed into the floor. If you're doing it right, you will feel the stretch pulling on the muscles in the backs of your lower legs. Hold this position for a count of 10, relax for a count of five, then hold again for 10.

"Hitting the wall" for some old-fashioned, sensible prevention three times a day should help you sleep better at night and keep your muscles in better, more limber shape.

Say 'nuts' to sore legs

If you suffer from pain and heaviness in your legs, you might find relief in the shape of a large brown nut from the horse chestnut tree. This seed contains a substance called aescin, which improves your body's circulation by strengthening the tone and condition of your veins.

When your veins are in good shape, your blood moves more smoothly between your heart and other parts of your body. So you're less likely to suffer varicose veins or fluid buildup — two problems that can cause painful, swollen legs.

Horse chestnut is a popular herbal remedy in Europe where the German Commission E, which is similar to our Food and Drug Administration, has approved it for treating leg pain and swelling, and problems such as varicose veins.

In one study, horse chestnut extract reduced lower leg swelling just as well as more traditional treatments such as compression stockings and diuretic drugs. The herb was found to be more convenient than compression and did not drain the body of other nutrients, as diuretics can.

Horse chestnut extract is available at health food stores. If you want to try it, see your doctor first to determine if your achy, swollen legs are symptoms of a more serious condition. They might be a red flag for liver or kidney problems, heart failure, or pregnancy.

Lung Cancer

Fight lung cancer with nutritional know-how

Even if you don't smoke, you can still get lung cancer. But experts say if you eat more fruits and vegetables and cut back on fat, you have a fighting chance to avoid this disease.

Carrots, especially, have a protective benefit against lung cancer, according to a study at the Karolinska Institute in Sweden. Researchers say that's because they are high in beta carotene, a nutrient your body converts into vitamin A. It's a powerful antioxidant that fights free radical damage in your body — the kind that causes cancer.

To get the most beta carotene in your diet, choose produce with deep, dark colors like these:

▶ Fruits — dried apricots, mango, cantaloupe, and pumpkin

▶ Vegetables — carrots, sweet potatoes, tomatoes, spinach, broccoli, collard greens, and parsley

If you find it hard to work foods like these into your menu, don't despair. While the National Cancer Institute recommends five servings of fruits and vegetables daily for maximum health, researchers have found that eating just one-and-a-half servings each day can reduce your risk of lung cancer by 40 percent. That's a big benefit from such a little effort.

And don't worry if you prefer your vegetables cooked instead of raw. Scientists are now saying it's OK to use that saucepan and casserole dish because cooked vegetables are not nearly as bad as they used to think. In a study comparing processed carrots and spinach to the same raw vegetables, people actually absorbed more healthy beta carotene from the processed vegetables.

While you're enjoying more fruits and vegetables, don't forget to go easy on the fatty foods. If your diet is loaded with saturated fat, you're five times as likely to develop lung cancer as a woman who eats little fat.

Learn to make low-fat choices — read labels, eat chicken or fish, and go for made-from-skim cheeses and other dairy products. You'll breathe easier knowing your healthy choices are helping your lungs, too.

Slash cancer risk with superstar mineral

A rather humble nutrient may play a starring role in the fight against lung cancer. A recent study by the National Public Health Institute in Finland found that you may be at higher risk for developing lung cancer if your body is low in selenium. Other studies have shown that this antioxidant trace mineral not only slashes your cancer risk but benefits almost every part of your body.

Don't rush out to buy selenium supplements, however, since few people in developed countries are deficient in this nutrient, and taking too much can be toxic. If you eat a normal diet with plenty of unprocessed foods, you should be fine. You'll find selenium in many grains, nuts, and vegetables; meat, especially organ meats like liver; and seafood.

Green tea — the answer to cancer?

Why do the Japanese have a lower rate of lung cancer than Americans even though they smoke nearly twice as many cigarettes? The answer might lie in the bottom of a small porcelain cup.

Green tea is the traditional beverage of many Eastern countries, including Japan, where the cancer rate is significantly lower than in the Western world. Scientists believe there is a connection.

Green tea (and to a lesser extent black tea) contains strong antioxidants called polyphenols that stop the growth and spread of malignant tumors and combat cancer that has already formed. They can even kill cancer cells without affecting healthy ones. That means if you have cancer, polyphenols can actually help you live longer.

There is convincing evidence that green tea not only protects against lung cancer but also a host of other cancers including skin, stomach, colon, breast, esophageal, gastrointestinal, liver, and pancreatic. Maybe the most encouraging news is that you can see positive effects no matter when you start drinking it. In some studies, the tea attacked the growth of stomach cancer even during the later stages of development.

Do you need to drink gallons of tea to reap any benefit? Experts say no. But they can't quite agree on a magic amount, since different studies have given different answers.

► Researchers at Purdue University say you need four cups a day to get enough of the anti-cancer compound to make a difference.

► Other studies say as little as one cup a week will slash your risk of developing cancer of the esophagus (the tube that carries food from your throat to your stomach) by as much as 50 percent. Drink green tea once a week for six months or more, and you'll have a 30-percent-lower risk of stomach cancer.

► If you really want to hedge your bets, a study from the Saitama Cancer Center Research Institute in Japan says drinking 10 cups a day can delay the onset of cancer by more than eight years in women and three years in men.

It may be confusing, but the bottom line is — even small amounts seem to help, so you'd be smart to work this beverage into your daily routine. If you find you don't like the taste, try supplements. Most health food stores carry green tea capsules containing standardized extracts of polyphenols, the antioxidants that give tea its healing powers.

You can also stick with black tea if you're used to drinking that. The leaves come from the same plant as green tea but are processed longer and allowed to ferment, which destroys some of the beneficial polyphenols. But researchers have found that this type of tea also reduces the risk of certain cancers.

Whatever type you choose, by taking time each day for a little "spot of tea," you'll enjoy a warm, relaxing way to better health.

Macular Degeneration

Fight eye disease with a rainbow of foods

Good eyesight makes you appreciate the beautiful colors of a rainbow and may even help you find the proverbial pot of gold. But your eyes will be richer if you find a pot of golden fruits and vegetables instead — and orange, red, and green ones, too.

Brightly colored foods that contain the carotenoids lutein and zeaxanthin can lower your risk of developing age-related macular degeneration by 43 percent. This eye condition is the leading cause of blindness in people over 65. So you'll want to ensure sharp eyesight by eating foods in those healthy hues.

Previous research touted leafy green vegetables as the best source of carotenoids to help protect against macular degeneration. However, a recent study found that corn has the highest percentage of lutein while orange peppers are your richest source of zeaxanthin. To get both of these carotenoids at once, eat some kiwi, red seedless grapes, or zucchini squash.

Or have an egg. It turns out egg yolk is actually the best source of both lutein and zeaxanthin. Researchers suggest that if you've given up eggs in the past, you might want to reconsider. Not only are they good for your eyes, but they may not be as harmful to the arteries as experts once thought. But to be on the safe side, if you increase the number of eggs you eat, you might want to cut out an equal amount of saturated fat somewhere else in your diet. Try eating less meat or whole dairy products.

The American Heart Association still recommends limiting your egg consumption to three or four per week. It's best not to cook them in fat. You can boil or poach them, or prepare them in a frying pan lightly coated with a nonfat spray.

Studies also show that antioxidant vitamins C and E and the mineral selenium may help protect your eyes from macular degeneration. Lycopene, another carotenoid found in abundance in tomato sauce, also had positive results in studies. Emphasize colorful fruits and vegetables in your diet, and you'll get a good supply of all these protective nutrients.

Menopause

Think 'natural' for a smooth transition

Menopause is sometimes referred to as the "change of life." Between the ages of 40 and 50, many women find that not only do their bodies change, but their personal and professional lives change as well.

Annoying symptoms, like insomnia or hot flashes, frequently come at the onset of menopause. They vary in intensity and gradually subside.

"Clearly not all women experience menopause alike," says registered pharmacist Constance Grauds of San Rafael, California. "While 75 to 80 percent of menopausal women experience one or more physical symptoms, only 10 to 35 percent are affected strongly enough to see their doctor."

In addition, potentially life-threatening conditions, like osteoporosis and heart disease, are waiting to ambush you. Some women choose to take hormones as a way to reduce these dangers. Others look for different ways to ease the transition because of side effects from HRT.

Hot flashes. Not every woman finds those sudden "power surges" uncomfortable. Grauds says, "If hot flashes are not bothersome to you, relax and enjoy the warmth, as they are not innately harmful to the body." But if you wish to avoid them, Grauds recommends eating lots of foods rich in calcium. Also include plenty of vitamin E from whole grains, cold-pressed oils, green leafy vegetables, and some nuts — almonds, for example. You may also want to avoid anything that heats up the body, like coffee, alcohol, and hot spices. And if you smoke, give that up, too. A recent study at the Baltimore Veterans Affairs Medical Center found that women who smoke have significantly more hot flashes than nonsmokers.

Excess water. If you avoid salty foods and drink more liquids, you may be able to prevent the bloating, tenderness, and depression that can come with water retention. Also, eat foods high in water content, such as melons, celery, and fruits. Drink natural herbal teas of cornsilk or dandelion leaf for their diuretic effect.

Vaginal dryness. Some women experience this problem for a year or so at the onset of menopause. It can be painful if the vaginal lining becomes inflamed. "You can help yourself naturally," says Grauds, "by eating foods high in vitamin E and drinking lots of liquids."

Insomnia. You can choose from a number of herbs to soothe yourself into slumber. For example, you might relax with a cup of valerian or passion flower tea. "Some women get relief from their insomnia with hops, chamomile, lemon balm, oat straw, catnip — even St. John's wort," says Grauds. You can find these as dried herbs, tinctures, or capsules.

Osteoporosis. Osteoporosis is a condition that possibly began when you were a teenager. During those adolescent years, you set yourself up for the quality of bone density you would have as a mature adult. Consider yourself fortunate if your mother made you drink lots of milk. That means stronger bones and a better chance of evading the crippling effects of osteoporosis. However, even if you didn't grow up drinking a lot of milk, all is not lost. You can begin strengthening your bones today. The key word is calcium.

The National Research Council has determined that a healthy pre-menopausal woman needs 1,000 to 1,200 mg of calcium a day. If you're postmenopausal, you need up to 1,500 mg of this bone-strengthening mineral. That's a lot of calcium for anyone. Of course, it's best to get it from natural sources: dairy foods, seafood such as oysters and sardines, and vegetables like kale and beet greens. But if you don't feel you can eat that much calcium, you can turn to supplements.

Because of the decrease in estrogen during menopause, you are probably going to gain weight. It's a sad fact for most women but simply your body's reaction to the change in hormones. Being more physically active will help you avoid this problem. Be careful about dieting at this time though. At least one study has shown that weight loss in postmenopausal women significantly increases bone loss, and that means a higher risk of osteoporosis.

Heart disease. During and after menopause, you are more at risk of developing heart disease than at any other time in your life. But by adjusting your diet, you can say goodbye to this concern and really enjoy your golden years.

Heart-healthy eating is simple — low fat, high fiber. But one study has shown that this advice probably should be modified for postmenopausal women. It seems that a high-carbohydrate, low-fat diet increases risk factors for heart disease in these women. Replacing saturated fat with the monounsaturated and polyunsaturated kind found in olive, canola, vegetable, and soybean oils may actually work better than adding more carbohydrates to your diet.

Enjoy caffeine in moderation

All you poor coffee-holics who simply have to have your morning cup, but agonize over the health risks, can now relax. A little. The old news from several studies was that drinking caffeine, especially more than two to three cups a day, caused bone loss in postmenopausal women if they took in less than 800 mg of calcium per day.

However, a new, more carefully controlled study did not find this to be true. Even those women who drank up to eight or more cups of coffee per day showed no changes in bone density. Of course, caffeine can affect you in other ways, so it's still best to limit your intake. If you are a healthy, postmenopausal woman who likes her morning cup of coffee, go ahead and enjoy it. But be sure to take the recommended amount of calcium, and switch off the coffee pot after breakfast.

Let the air out of hot flashes

Most women have been conditioned to think "stomach in, chest out" from the time they were young girls aiming to attract a few admiring glances. But if you are dealing with the discomforts of menopause, you're probably more interested in cooling down your hot flashes than heating up the opposite sex.

So now it's time to "let it all hang out," as they say. Pushing out your abdomen, instead of holding it in, will give you more room to breathe deeply. And that, researchers say, may be the key to blocking those "power surges."

"We've done three published studies on slow, deep breathing, and the flash frequency decreases by about 50 percent," says psychologist Robert Freedman of Detroit's Wayne State University School of Medicine. And he adds, "There are no bad side effects." This is good news if you can't or don't want to use hormone treatment to lessen menopause symptoms.

According to Dr. Freedman, the women in his studies learned how to slow their breathing to half their usual rate. "We train them in eight weekly sessions about one hour each and tell them to practice twice a day for 15 minutes," says Freedman. "Later, when they're in a situation where they're likely to get a flash, like a hot room, they do the deep, slow breathing."

If you're experiencing the red face and drenching sweat of hot flashes, this "belly breathing" technique may be just what you need. To practice it:

- ▶ Lie on your back with the palms of your hands flat against your abdomen, middle fingers almost touching.

- ▶ Breathe in slowly through your nose, keeping your chest still, but letting your stomach expand. The fingers will separate as you inhale. Continue breathing in until your abdomen reaches a comfortably full feeling.

- ▶ Slowly begin to exhale, also through your nose. Allow the muscles of your abdomen to pull back in, pushing the air out. You'll notice that the fingers now move back closer together.

When you get comfortable with how belly breathing feels lying down, practice it while sitting and standing up. That way, you'll be able to use it no matter where you are. Before you know it, you'll be ready to blow those hot flashes away.

4 unique ways to chase away symptoms

"Post-menopausal zest!" That's how anthropologist Margaret Mead described the renewed energy that many women experience when their menstrual periods stop. As you reach the change of life, chances are you'll find it's not as physically and emotionally distressing as you feared.

In a national survey of over 3,000 adults, the post-menopausal women were asked how they felt when their menstrual periods stopped completely. A surprising 62 percent said they felt only relief. Another 25 percent reported having no particular feeling about it, while a mere 2 percent said they felt only regret at reaching this stage of life. The rest, about 11 percent, had mixed feelings.

The peri-menopausal women — those in the process of the menstrual changes — and those who were premenopausal were asked how they think they'll feel when their periods stop.

"The major difference by menopausal stage was that peri- and premenopausal women were more apt to have mixed feelings than post-menopausal women," said Dr. Alice Rossi of the University of Massachusetts, one of the researchers.

In the survey, sponsored by the MacArthur Foundation, both men and women were asked questions about symptoms related to menopause and aging. You'll probably find their responses encouraging.

"Irritability was not related to menopausal phase. It's age related, decreasing the older the person gets — man or woman," says Rossi.

And only 30 percent of the women reported having hot flashes as often as once a week, even between ages 50 and 55, the peak years for symptoms during the menopausal transition.

Rossi analyzed the results of the study to learn what predicts whether a woman experiences high or low levels of menopausal symptoms. You might use what she found to minimize your own discomforts as you approach the change of life.

▶ **Stay healthy.** Women who rated their physical and mental health as poor or moderate had more problems with symptoms than those who reported their health as excellent.

▶ **Reduce stress.** "High levels of stress in their family roles," says Rossi, "trigger elevated symptoms scores for both sexes."

▶ **Continue learning.** Those who were better educated suffered fewer symptoms. If you've always wanted to go back to school, this may be a good time to go.

▶ **Work on your self-image.** "I asked women to rate the extent to which they think their bodies have changed ... in terms of energy, physical fitness, physique or figure, and weight," says Rossi. She found more symptoms reported by those who felt they were "worse now than five years ago."

If you have had a lot of problems with menstruation, pay special attention to these suggestions. Rossi noticed that women who experienced a lot of discomfort with their monthly periods were more likely to find the same with menopause.

Mitral Valve Prolapse Syndrome

8 simple remedies ease frustrating condition

Linda was lying quietly in bed, trying to sleep, when her heart began to pound. "I felt as if it was going to jump right out of my chest. I could actually see it beating through my clothes," she says. Trying to fight her rising panic just made the pounding worse. Was she having a heart attack? Was she going crazy? Finally her heart calmed down, and she fell asleep, exhausted. The next morning, she was so tired she could hardly drag herself out of bed.

If this scene sounds familiar, you may be suffering from mitral valve prolapse syndrome (MVPS). And relieving your frightening symptoms may be as simple as drinking more water, quitting caffeine, and getting a little more exercise.

Doctors have known for years that some people have a floppy valve in their hearts that allows some blood to flow back into the upper chamber of the heart. This "prolapse" can be heard through a stethoscope as a clicking sound, sometimes along with a murmur. It's more common than you may think. As many as one out of every 10 people may have this condition.

But you can have this leaky heart valve and not be bothered by such frightening symptoms as chest pain, heart palpitations, dizziness, extreme fatigue, and panic attacks. Doctors now think these and other minor symptoms are caused by a nervous system disorder, called dysautonomia, that affects your body's basic functions.

"It's really not a cardiac problem, so mitral valve prolapse syndrome is probably not a good name for it," says Dr. Phillip Watkins, head of the Mitral Valve Prolapse Center in Birmingham, Alabama.

Watkins says one problem that results from dysautonomia is low blood volume, meaning your body doesn't have as much fluid as it's supposed to. "If you take a patient with prolapse, dump out all the fluid from her arteries and veins, it's only about 80 percent of what it should be," he says. He believes low blood volume is a major cause of most of the troubling symptoms of this condition.

To test for low blood volume, Watkins recommends having your blood pressure checked two ways, while seated and then immediately after standing. If your pressure plunges when you stand, your blood volume may be too low.

If you do have MVPS, your doctor may prescribe medicine to control the symptoms that affect your heart. But before you consider medication, try making some changes in your lifestyle. These steps can make a huge difference in the way you feel.

Drink lots of water. Watkins believes this is the most critical step of all. By drinking at least eight glasses of water a day (64 ounces), you'll keep your blood volume high and help relieve your symptoms.

Get more salt in your diet. You don't want to go overboard on salt, but eating a few more salty foods will keep more fluid in your body. This should help prevent low blood pressure, dizziness, and the feeling that you are going to faint.

Follow a healthy diet. An unbalanced diet full of junk food will contribute to your fatigue.

Quit caffeine. That power punch of caffeine in coffee, tea, and colas is a drug that stimulates your nervous system. Additional stimulation of your nervous system is not what you need — it will throw things even more out of balance.

Eat less sugar. When you eat something packed with sugar, it causes your blood glucose to shoot up, and this stimulates your autonomic nervous system. If you're feeling tired and want a snack to give you a little energy, a healthy one that contains some protein is a better choice.

Get enough magnesium. Medical studies have shown a connection between magnesium deficiency and the symptoms of MVPS. Most people don't get enough of this mineral because their diets are high in processed foods. Avocados, sunflower seeds, pinto beans, black-eyed peas, raw almonds, green leafy vegetables, and whole, mostly unprocessed, cereal grains are good sources of magnesium. Talk with your doctor before taking any magnesium in supplement form. Too much can be harmful.

Exercise. With the fatigue that accompanies MVPS, you probably don't feel much like exercising. But exercise is one of the most important tools for keeping your heart healthy and your autonomic nervous system in balance. Start with mild aerobic exercise then work your way up to more intense activity as you begin to feel better.

Avoid triggers. Skipping meals or getting tired and stressed out can strain your health and worsen the signs of MVPS. So can alcohol, smoking, illness such as a cold or flu, menstruation, menopause, and even being in a hot, dry environment. Some over-the-counter cold and sinus medications contain stimulants that can make your symptoms worse, so check the labels.

Although this condition is not life threatening, it can wreak havoc with your daily routine. Knowing how to manage your symptoms is the key to getting your life back to normal. As Linda says, "The more you know about mitral valve prolapse syndrome, the better. Being educated about it is the best way to deal with it, and to live with it."

For more information, contact the National Dysautonomia Research Foundation at 1407 W. Fourth Street, Suite 160, Red Wing, MN 55066-2108 or online at <www.ndrf.org>.

Guard your heart from a deadly bug

If you have mitral valve prolapse and you're planning to visit the dentist, make sure you mention your condition beforehand. Your dentist, or doctor, may need to prescribe an antibiotic to help you avoid a rare bacterial infection called endocarditis.

Any kind of dental work that causes bleeding, including cleanings, might give you a serious infection that will inflame the lining of your heart valves. This condition can be fatal if not treated. Taking an antibiotic before your dental procedure prevents the bacteria from taking hold in your heart.

This also applies if you are having surgery or a medical test in which bacteria might enter your bloodstream. Check with your doctor to see if she thinks you might need an antibiotic before the procedure. A little advance preparation can help you avoid this potentially deadly disease.

Night Blindness

Choose the blues for sharper sight

Blueberries, huckleberries, bilberries, or whortleberries — whatever you call your favorite in this family of fruits — their dusky skins hold the secret to seeing better in the dark.

For many years people in Europe have praised bilberries for a variety of health reasons, including improvements to their eyesight. British pilots during World War II ate bilberry jam to help them see better when flying night missions.

Canadian food chemist Wilhelmina Kalt, PhD, credits the pigments — called anthocyanins — for the benefits. That's what gives the intense dark blue color to all the blueberry cousins. These pigments are powerful antioxidants that counteract the damage free radicals do to the body.

"Most red and purple fruits have anthocyanins," says Kalt. "The content varies. But all the blueberries have a lot more anthocyanins than most other fruits that are available in North America — like raspberries and strawberries, for example."

Eat bilberries for better eyesight. Kalt has found in her studies that of all the fruits in the blueberry family, the bilberry has the highest amount of anthocyanins. And so far, it's the only one you can buy as a supplement.

Although people take it for different reasons, a main benefit seems to be the sharper eyesight. "In my personal experience talking with people," says Kalt, "what those taking bilberry supplements notice most is a difference in visual acuity."

And research shows that people who depend on good night vision — air traffic controllers, pilots, and truck drivers — do, indeed, see better at night when they take bilberry supplements. They find it helps them adjust to darkness more quickly. And it helps them bounce back from the effects of flashes of light — like from the bright headlights of an on-coming car.

Reap the benefits of blueberries. The most potent blueberry seems to be the lowbush variety that grows wild in Maine and eastern Canada. Kalt points out their advantage over highbush blueberries that grow farther south.

"The wild, or lowbush, blueberry," she says, "is higher, pound for pound, in anthocyanin content than the larger, plumper highbush blueberries." That's because they are smaller and have more skin per ounce. Since anthocyanins are found in the skin of the fruit, you reap more antioxidant benefits.

Their shelf life is short, however, so unless you live in the region where wild blueberries grow, you probably won't find fresh ones. But supermarkets have them frozen, canned, or in prepared products like muffins or jams, all year long.

The benefits of blueberries don't stop with their antioxidant protection. They're also low in calories — about 80 per cup — and high in vitamins and fiber. And there are plenty of ways to enjoy them. Munch some blueberry pie, pancakes, and waffles. Sprinkle a few on your morning cereal. Stir them into a cup of yogurt, or blend a healthy fruit smoothie. You'll be doing your body — especially your eyes — a great favor.

Improve your night vision

After age 50, most people find it gets harder to see contrasts. This can make driving in the dark especially difficult and frustrating. But a new contact lens could brighten your outlook.

Professor Josef Bille of Heidelberg University in Germany has developed a new lens that helps correct the refractive error around your pupil. He says that will help you see contrasts at least five times better. You'll benefit most by wearing the lenses at night, but they can help whenever you have a problem distinguishing contrasts.

The lenses will be sold as daily disposables, but you may have to wait a couple of years before you find them on the market.

Osteoporosis

Fight bone loss with these nutritional 'secrets'

You may think you know everything you need to know about osteoporosis. You've been bombarded for years with the facts, the tips, the latest studies, the latest diets. You know you need to keep your bones strong and healthy. You know it affects lots of people — more than 200 million throughout the world. You know it's the major cause of bone fractures in seniors.

But there are some things about osteoporosis you may not know. Like the fact that about 20 percent of those with the disease are men. Or that most people think they are getting plenty of calcium in their diet — but they're wrong.

Here's some news you can use to help keep your bones strong.

Add some variety. The National Academy of Science set 1,200 milligrams (mg) of calcium every day as the recommended dietary allowance (RDA) for people over 50. You're probably thinking, "That's a lot of milk — about three and a half cups. And I don't even like milk that much." The fact is, dairy products aren't the only good, absorbable sources of calcium.

Dr. Ann Hunt, Associate Professor of Nursing at Purdue University, says there are several other sources that many people don't know about. "Canned sardines and salmon with bones in them are great ways to get calcium in your diet. And the bones are kind of tasty and crunchy." Other bone-building foods are enriched orange juice, oysters, nuts, chickpeas, broccoli, tofu, navy beans, soybeans, collards, and turnip greens. Hunt cautions, "But don't try to get your calcium from just one of these sources. You would need to eat a huge amount of broccoli, for instance, to achieve your daily requirement. Instead, eat a wide variety of fruits and vegetables."

Toss a salad. Whenever you think about osteoporosis, you naturally think of calcium. But there are other nutrients just as important to good bone health, like magnesium, B6, and vitamin K.

Researchers at Harvard Medical School found that vitamin K deficiencies are linked to brittle bones and high fracture rates. They studied one food, in particular, containing vitamin K that really made a difference in bone density — iceberg lettuce. This humble, leafy green, which has become less popular than more exotic types of lettuce, is an easy, healthy way to fight osteoporosis.

In the Harvard study, women who ate a cup of lettuce, which contains about 146 micrograms (mcg) of vitamin K, at least once a day lowered their risk of hip fracture by 45 percent. Although the RDA for vitamin K is only 90 mcg for women over 50 and 120 mcg for men over 50, this study urges people at risk to get at least 100 mcg of vitamin K a day. Experts warn that natural food sources of vitamin K, like lettuce, are fine, but if you are currently taking aspirin or another anticoagulant to fight blood clots, talk with your doctor before taking a vitamin K supplement.

In general, what experts have found is that if you're not getting enough calcium, it's likely you're not getting enough of several other important nutrients. Try to get as many vitamins and minerals as you can through whole foods. Use supplements only if you can't get enough in your diet.

Enjoy some soy. Tofu, TVP, tempeh, miso — not your ordinary shopping list, but if you're concerned about osteoporosis, you might add some of these soy products to your pantry.

Soy protein, which comes from soybeans, is rich in bone-building calcium and isoflavones. Several studies have proven that including soy protein in your diet can increase your bones' density. Although soy doesn't seem to be able to reverse the effects of osteoporosis, it may prevent them.

Medical interest in soy was first sparked when scientists discovered how little osteoporosis occurs in Eastern countries, like China and Japan, where soy makes up a large part of the diet.

Although lower in fat, especially saturated fat, than most animal proteins, soybeans still contain 19 percent polyunsaturated fat. To keep those fat grams under control, look for low-fat soy products, like low-fat soy milk and tofu, and replace high-fat, low-fiber meats with soy-based foods. Don't just add soy products to a typical high-protein American diet. That can lead to kidney trouble.

Be aware that many experts are concerned about the connection between soy and forgetfulness discovered several years ago. The research suggests soy makes your brain age faster. While you don't have to avoid soy altogether, talk to your doctor about keeping to moderate amounts.

Be on the lookout for a man-made version of the bone-saving isoflavone found naturally in soy. Called ipriflavone, this supplement gives your body the benefits of estrogen without any of the negative side effects. It prevents bone thinning, but it doesn't cause tissue growth that can lead to breast or uterine cancer.

Beware of certain foods. Some substances in food will actually keep your body from absorbing and using the calcium your bones need to stay strong and healthy. Fiber, especially from bran and high-fiber fruits and vegetables, and oxalate, found in cranberries, chard, rhubarb, spinach, and beet leaves, are two of the culprits. Don't stop eating these nutritious foods. Just make sure you eat plenty of high-calcium foods, like eggs, beans, or milk, along with them to offset their negative effects.

Protein and sodium increase the amount of calcium your body gets rid of through your urine. So lowering the amount of both protein and sodium in your diet may help you keep more of the calcium you take in.

And if you're a coffee drinker, the caffeine in one cup of coffee can increase your daily need for calcium by 30 to 50 mg.

Keeping fit means stronger bones

After you turn 35, your body can't rebuild bones the way it used to, but you can slow down the process that drains calcium — and strength — from them.

Many experts think weight-bearing exercises are a good way to do this. These exercises, which make you work against gravity, keep your bones from deteriorating, as proven by the space program. Scientists say astronauts lose bone mass in space, an environment without gravity, up to 10 times faster than on Earth.

Weight-bearing exercises include strength training, stair-climbing, hiking, jogging, walking, and dancing. Activities like swimming and cycling are great for your heart and lungs, but they don't slow down bone loss.

In one study, postmenopausal women who didn't normally exercise began strength-training exercises twice a week. After one year, their bone density had improved to the point they were able to function as if they were 15 to 20 years younger.

Dr. Ann Hunt, Associate Professor of Nursing at Purdue University, warns, "Weight-bearing exercises, like walking, are good, but they don't benefit your arms. And there are lots of osteoporotic fractures of the arms — wrists, especially. So you need to do some weight-bearing on your arms. Now that doesn't mean bench-pressing 300 pounds. It means doing some exercises with cans of tomatoes or even sacks of rice." You need a good, well-rounded workout, but you don't have to go to a gym in order to get it.

Another great exercise program for seniors is called Pilates — a combination of yoga and strength training.

It gives you the benefits of stretching and improved balance, along with better muscle tone and increased strength. Look for a Pilates class in your community.

And don't forget one of the most natural forms of exercise — sex. Dr. Joel D. Block, who wrote *Secrets of Better Sex*, says that having regular sex causes your body to produce more estrogen than normal. This is a plus for your bones and also your heart, especially as you move into menopause.

Talk with your doctor before starting an exercise program if you are over 40, already have osteoporosis, or have any other health problems. And use common sense. Start slowly, increase your activity gradually, and never try to exercise through any pain or discomfort.

Depression raises risk of osteoporosis

If you've ever suffered from real, down-in-the-dumps depression, you may have a higher risk of developing osteoporosis.

Scientists are still trying to pinpoint the connection, but many think it has something to do with the hormone cortisol. When people are depressed, their adrenal glands go into overtime and produce too much cortisol, which can cause your bones to thin and lose density.

Other factors related to depression could also contribute to osteoporosis, like not eating right and getting any exercise. And if your doctor has prescribed medication to treat your depression, ask him about side effects. Several drugs used to treat depression can cause bone loss.

How to get the most from calcium supplements

One of the most common questions Dr. Ann Hunt, Associate Professor of Nursing at Purdue University, gets asked is, "What about supplements?" According to Hunt, not all calcium supplements are created equal, and they work best under specific conditions. Here are some things you should do if you decide to use a supplement.

Check absorption. Most professionals are concerned with how much calcium actually gets into your bloodstream where it can do your bones some good. This is called absorption. Sometimes the calcium from supplements doesn't make it into your system. The supplement just sits in your stomach, without dissolving.

To test whether or not your body will break down and absorb a calcium supplement, place the tablet in 6 ounces of vinegar or warm water. Let it sit for about 30 minutes, stirring occasionally. If it's still not completely dissolved after half an hour, it probably won't dissolve in your stomach, either.

Take small doses. Since calcium isn't absorbed very well, Hunt advises taking several small supplemental doses throughout the day.

"If you take a huge amount of calcium," she says, "only a small percentage is absorbed anyway."

Eat when you supplement. For best absorption, take calcium supplements with food. Hunt explains, "Hydrochloric acid in your stomach helps break down and digest your food. As you get older, your stomach just normally produces less. However, when you eat, your stomach produces extra acid, which then breaks down the calcium." Experts say calcium absorption increases by about 10 percent when taken with food.

Choose wisely. There's a great deal of controversy over which kind of supplement is better — calcium carbonate or calcium citrate. The truth is, Hunt says, they both have pros and cons. "Calcium carbonate is more easily absorbed, but it causes a lot of gastric distress, such as bloating. Calcium citrate doesn't cause as many intestinal problems but less of it is absorbed. That means you need to take more of the calcium citrate to get your minimum calcium requirements." Read the label for how much of the supplement is absorbable calcium and make a dosage decision you're comfortable with.

Watch your D. Vitamin D plays an important role in how much calcium your bones actually absorb. Studies have proven that low levels of vitamin D go hand-in-hand with weaker, more fragile bones. That's why experts suggest taking vitamin D with your calcium supplements to help reduce your risk of bone fractures. Hunt says, "You can certainly take too much vitamin D and get into other problems, but 400 to 800 international units (IU) a day is about right."

Your body manufactures vitamin D when exposed to sunshine, but during the winter you are exposed to less sunshine and may experience more bone loss. In addition, sunscreens will block some of your body's absorption of this important vitamin. You don't need to sunbathe in January or give up your sunscreen — just make sure you take in vitamin D from good nutritional sources each day. Fortified milk is the richest food source of vitamin D. You can also find it in other fortified dairy products and cereals; egg yolks; liver; and fatty fish, like salmon, tuna, and sardines.

Build your bones with chocolate

Chocolate lovers now have a reason to splurge without feeling guilty. A new candy-like product, called Viactiv Soft Calcium Chews, can satisfy your chocolate craving and strengthen your bones, too. Each chew contains 500 milligrams (mg) of calcium, which is half the daily requirement for a premenopausal woman, as well as vitamins D and K to help your body absorb the calcium. Eating two squares a day is a sweet way to get the extra calcium your body needs.

Just be sure you don't overindulge, especially if you are taking aspirin or some other anticoagulant regularly. Too much vitamin K can interfere with these blood thinners.

Ovarian Cancer

Delicious way to dodge ovarian cancer

When you're at the grocery store, do you wander down the aisles trying to decide what to have for dinner? If you're a woman over 35, make sure the menu includes broccoli or carrots and a little cabbage. These vegetables may lower your risk of developing ovarian cancer, the fourth leading cause of cancer-related deaths.

The American Cancer Society estimates that about 25,000 new cases of ovarian cancer are diagnosed each year, and half of these cancer victims will die.

Although there's still no proven way to prevent ovarian cancer, eating certain foods might help reduce your risk.

Studies have shown that beta carotene, an antioxidant found in dark green and dark orange fruits and vegetables, can protect against ovarian cancer. Carrots topped the list as offering the most protection.

Another important antioxidant is the mineral selenium. If you want to improve your odds against ovarian cancer, make sure you eat selenium-rich foods, like seafood, grains, and vegetables. Researchers at Johns Hopkins University in Maryland found that high levels of selenium were associated with a lower risk of ovarian cancer.

Vegetables in the cabbage family — including brussels sprouts, kale, and cauliflower — may also offer some protection.

You've known for years about the many benefits of eating fruits and vegetables. This just gives you another reason to add them to your shopping list.

Latest risk for breast cancer survivors

Researchers have suspected a connection between breast cancer and ovarian cancer for many years, and it seems they were right. A recent study at the University of California, Irvine, confirms that women who had breast cancer before age 50 are at greater risk for ovarian cancer.

Ovarian cancer is very difficult to diagnose. Tests to detect it are unreliable, and the symptoms are vague. These symptoms include discomfort or swelling in your lower abdomen, feeling full after eating very little, loss of appetite, gas and indigestion, nausea, weight loss, frequent urination, constipation, and pain during sexual intercourse.

Besides being a breast cancer survivor, other risk factors for ovarian cancer include a personal history of colon or endometrial cancer, a family history of ovarian cancer, never having children, age, and obesity. Taking birth control pills, having at least one full-term pregnancy, and breast-feeding reduces the risk.

If you have any of the risk factors for ovarian cancer, talk with your doctor. He can help you decide what screening methods are appropriate for you, and he'll know what to look for during your yearly examination.

Prostate Cancer

Shield yourself from this slow-growing killer

It has been said that more men will die *with* prostate cancer than *from* it. This is because it tends to affect older men and is typically a slow-growing cancer. So even if you get it, you're likely to die from other causes before the cancer gets bad enough to kill you.

Nevertheless, prostate cancer claims about 42,000 lives a year, and men probably fear it more than almost any other disease. But there are ways to shield yourself from this form of cancer, and one of the best ways is to change your eating habits.

Get vitamin and mineral protection. You need the right balance of vitamins and minerals to have an overall healthy body. But which ones are most important to prostate health? Vitamin E is a powerful antioxidant that may help fight prostate cancer by preventing free-radical damage to your DNA. In a recent study, men who took 50 mg of vitamin E daily were 32 percent less likely to suffer symptoms of prostate cancer. Natural sources of vitamin E include wheat germ, almonds, peanuts, and sunflower seeds.

Studies find that vitamin D, the sunshine vitamin, also may inhibit prostate cancer, which may be why men who live in Southern climates are less likely to get the disease. The trace mineral selenium is another nutrient you want to get enough of. A large study at Harvard recently found that men with the highest intake of selenium were less likely to get prostate cancer than men with the lowest intake. You can find selenium in grains, shellfish, poultry, garlic, and egg yolks.

Limit fat. Men who eat a lot of fat, especially saturated fat, are asking for trouble. If you take in more than 35 grams of saturated fat per day, you have a 60 percent greater risk of prostate cancer.

Saturated fats are found mainly in animal products like dairy and red meat, so they may be among your favorite foods. Although you don't have to give those foods up completely, you should limit your fat intake to no more than 30 percent of your total calories, keeping saturated fat to only 10 percent.

Try more tomatoes. If you love pizza and spaghetti, you may be in luck. A Harvard study found the risk of prostate cancer was reduced by 45 percent among men who ate at least 10 servings of tomato-based products a week. Pizza, tomatoes, and tomato sauce were the three top prostate protectors. Researchers believe the substance responsible for this protective effect is lycopene, a carotenoid which gives tomatoes their red color.

Fill up on fiber. According to the National Cancer Institute, most people need to double their amount of daily fiber. It recommends 20 to 30 grams a day instead of the 11 grams the average person takes in. Evidence shows that a healthy intake of fiber may help prevent several types of cancer, including prostate cancer. One recent study found that a high intake of grains, cereals, and nuts was associated with a lower risk of prostate cancer.

Seek out soy. Hormone-related cancers like prostate and breast cancers cause far fewer deaths in the Far East than in the United States. That could be because Asians tend to eat more soy products like tofu, tempeh, soy sauce, soy milk, miso, and textured vegetable protein. Researchers believe that isoflavones, which are a type of phytoestrogen (estrogen-like compounds found in plants), are responsible for the soybean's protective effect.

One study found that soy sauce acted as an antioxidant, preventing the growth of cancer. Several components of soy sauce reduced stomach tumors in rats by 66 percent. And a recent study on Seventh-Day Adventists found that drinking soy milk more than once a day resulted in a 70 percent reduction in risk of prostate cancer.

Gulp some green tea. Another part of the Asian diet that may protect against prostate cancer is green tea. Several studies have found that green tea may help prevent several forms of cancers. In one test tube study, researchers found that a powerful antioxidant in green tea killed prostate cancer cells in both mice and humans, yet left healthy cells unharmed.

Although changing your diet to include prostate-healthy foods is no guarantee you'll avoid cancer, it will at least give you a good start. So load up on the fruits, vegetables, and grains, and go light on high-fat meat and dairy products, and you'll help your prostate stay healthy for years to come.

New test detects cancer early

Early detection of cancer sometimes means the difference between life and death. Now researchers have developed a new test that can detect a single telltale cell in a sample of blood. This could enable doctors to discover cancer in its earliest stages when it is most treatable.

The test uses magnets to detect epithelial cells. These are cells that are present in skin and other tissues but usually don't show up in your bloodstream. However, certain types of tumors, including breast and prostate tumors, are known to shed these cells as they develop, depositing the cells in your bloodstream.

Researchers studied blood samples from 30 people with breast cancer, three people with prostate cancer, and 13 cancer-free people. They discovered that the healthy people had only 1.5 epithelial cells per sample, while those with breast cancer showed a tremendous increase.

People with cancer that hadn't yet spread averaged 15.9 cells per sample, while those whose cancer had spread locally had an average of 47.4 cells. Subjects whose cancer had already invaded other parts of their bodies averaged a high of 122 epithelial cells.

Although more study is needed, scientists are hopeful this test will not only detect cancer earlier than is now possible, but also help track its progress and measure the success of treatments.

How to find the best doctor

You wouldn't look in the yellow pages for your future wife or husband, would you? You probably shouldn't use that method to find a new doctor, either. Choosing a doctor could be as important to your future as choosing a spouse, particularly when you're faced with a serious disease like cancer. The patient/doctor relationship is one on which your very life could hinge, so take the time to make an informed decision.

Hal Alpiar, author of *Doctor Shopping: How to Choose the Right Doctor for You and Your Family,* says having a list when you look for a doctor is even more important than having one for grocery shopping. Without a grocery list, you end up spending too much money and forgetting the items you really need. The same thing can happen when you shop for a doctor.

Your first step is to make a list of potential doctors that you can interview. You may have to pay for this interview time, but the investment will buy you a better sense of confidence and trust. Here are some suggestions on how to find the most qualified doctors.

Ask your current doctor. If you have a doctor you trust, ask him for recommendations. But keep in mind that he may have more than your best interests at heart.

"Be careful about taking doctor referrals from other doctors," Alpiar says. "A doctor may refer another doctor because they play golf together, share a vacation condo, or because the other doctor is a renowned researcher (perhaps with limited clinical experience)."

Alpiar also warns that hospital and other referral "services" are highly subjective because they only include those doctors who are affiliated with them, or who pay to be affiliated. "In other words, referral services that sound like objective resources very often are not," he says. "They are very often paid forms of advertising masquerading as public service programs."

Seek word-of-mouth recommendations. Ask your friends and family about their doctors and whether they've been happy with the care they've received. Keep in mind, however, that one person could be pleased as punch with a particular doctor, while another could be extremely dissatisfied. As with many things in life, much depends on the point of view. But if many people recommend the same doctor, your decision could be an easy one.

Focus on credentials. Look for a doctor who is board certified, particularly when searching for a specialist. This means that he has completed a training program and passed an extensive exam in his particular specialty. Most doctors today are board certified, so if yours isn't, he may not have passed the exam or hasn't taken the time to take the required classes in his specialty. Either way, you might want to consider another doctor.

To verify whether your doctor is board certified, check your library for the American Medical Association's Directory of Physicians. It contains information regarding each doctor's medical education, board certifications, licensing information, and any disciplinary actions taken against him. You can also call the American Board of Medical Specialties Hotline at 1-866-275-2267, or visit its website at <http://www.certifieddoctor.com/verify.html>.

Be prepared. When you visit a doctor you've decided to interview, take your list of questions with you. Make sure you include everything you're concerned about, even things you think are silly or embarrassing.

Write down the answers the doctor gives you, and don't be afraid to interrupt if you need to. Ask how many cases like yours she normally handles, and request examples, diagrams, similar experiences, and costs. Check on her certification and whether she has special training in your particular type of situation. But Alpiar warns, "Be aware that having a 'special interest' in a specific area of medicine or surgery does not necessarily make the doctor a specialist or expert any more than having a special interest in home runs makes someone a Mark McGwire."

Other issues to consider when choosing a doctor:

▶ **Convenience.** Is the doctor's office easy to get to? While this shouldn't be your primary consideration (a good doctor is worth a little drive time), being able to get to your doctor's office quickly and easily does make a difference to most people.

▶ **Office staff.** Are the receptionist and nurses professional and courteous? Often, the office staff reflects the attitude of the doctor.

▶ **Time.** Did you spend a lot of time reading magazines in the waiting room? It's understandable that a doctor sometimes gets tied up with a difficult case, and you have to wait. If it happens often, though, it could be a sign that the doctor regularly overbooks and may not have the time to give you the attention you deserve.

▶ **Attitude.** Was the doctor friendly, attentive, and willing to answer questions? Even if a doctor is competent and knowledgeable, if he rushes you in and out or seems distracted, you're not getting quality care. You deserve a doctor who will listen carefully to you and make decisions about your care that you are comfortable with.

The bottom line is, the more responsible you are for your own medical care, the better off you'll be. "In the end, it's your body that's being poked, prodded and prescribed to ... so take the responsibility that goes with that," Alpiar advises. "And find a doctor who's willing to be a 'partner' with you in health care."

―――――――

How to tell an O.D. from a D.O.

Are you confused by all those initials that follow your health-care provider's name? Just what do all those letters mean, and what do they mean to your health? Knowing what your doctor's credentials are can go a long way toward helping you make a decision on choosing a health-care provider that you're comfortable with.

- **Doctor of medicine (M.D.)** — These doctors can provide all types of medical care, including prescribing medicine and some surgery. They complete medical school, plus three to seven years of advanced medical education, and must be licensed by the state in which they practice.
- **Doctor of osteopathic medicine (D.O.)** — Osteopaths receive training similar to medical doctors and can

provide general health care, but they usually emphasize movement and manipulation in treating bone, joint, and muscle problems.

- **Psychologist (Ph.D., Psy.D., Ed.D., or M.A.)** — Psychologists are trained to treat people with mental and emotional disorders. They provide counseling but cannot prescribe medication. That responsibility falls to psychiatrists, who are medical doctors.

- **Optometrist (O.D.)** — Optometrists are trained to diagnose eye disorders and prescribe eyeglasses and contact lenses. In most states, they can also prescribe medicines to treat eye disorders but may refer patients to ophthalmologists, who are M.D.s, for problems that require surgery or medication.

- **Dentist (D.D.S. or D.M.D.)** — Dentists treat conditions of the mouth such as cavities and gum disease. They can prescribe medication and perform surgery on your mouth. Your dentist may refer you to another dental specialist, such as an oral surgeon (tooth extractions and surgery), an endodontist (root canals), or a periodontist (gum disease).

Raynaud's Phenomenon

Natural ways to beat cold hands and feet

Building a snowman, snow skiing, or taking a walk on a clear, cold night are activities that make winter delightful. If you have Raynaud's phenomenon (RP), however, just getting cold can turn into an extended bout with pain. Any exposure to frigid temperatures can bring a stinging and numbness to your hands and feet.

"Even something as simple as filling glasses with ice for a family dinner becomes a real problem for me," says 23-year-old Jennifer, who was diagnosed with Raynaud's five years ago. "After grabbing just a few ice cubes, my hands turn white, then a bluish color, then red. My hands feel numb, and then the pain starts."

This extreme sensitivity to cold affects about 10 percent of the population, usually women between the ages of 15 and 50. Raynaud's may strike out of the blue or stem from an underlying condition such as atherosclerosis, lupus, or rheumatoid arthritis. If you work with vibrating machinery, play the piano frequently, or have carpal tunnel syndrome, you're even more at risk. Oddly enough, it's not just the cold that provokes a painful reaction — emotional stress can do it as well.

Prevention is your best weapon in fighting this condition. Follow these tips to lessen your chances of suffering painful fingers and toes.

Bundle up. Medical studies in Great Britain have shown that body temperatures in Raynaud's sufferers drop faster than normal. It also takes them longer to get warm again. That's why it's important to protect yourself from cold at all times. Wear a warm coat, hat, gloves, and boots when you are outside in cold weather. Inside, protect yourself from cold drafts by snuggling in a warm blanket or quilt and wearing socks and shoes or slippers all the time.

Wear gloves in the house. Protect your hands whenever you take a package of frozen food from the freezer or fruit from the vegetable drawer. Keep a pair of clean winter gloves in the kitchen, along with potholders and towels you can fold around cold items while you take out the contents. Jennifer is always careful to wrap several layers of paper towels around a glass of cold water or a chilled soft drink before picking it up. Insulated drink holders made of Styrofoam are also helpful.

Pamper your pinkies. Keep your hands clean and dry, and try to keep them safe from cuts, scrapes, and bruises. Don't treat them roughly. If you develop any sores on your hands that don't heal, see your doctor.

Turn up the heat with pepper. Spicy cayenne pepper has a pain-relieving and warming effect on your skin. Sprinkle a little into your socks or gloves before you put them on to keep your hands and feet warmer. But first make sure you have no cuts or scrapes on your skin. Wash your hands thoroughly when you take off your gloves, and be careful not to touch your eyes or nose.

Cut out caffeine. This common drug affects your circulation and can have a negative effect on Raynaud's phenomenon. This includes the caffeine in coffee, tea, chocolate, and cola drinks, and many cold and cough remedies that contain decongestants.

Give ginkgo a go. Ginkgo is an ancient herbal remedy for improving your circulation. It may help your blood vessels stay open to improve blood flow in your fingers and toes. You can buy ginkgo as a food supplement in pill form in health food or discount stores.

Keep your environment smoke-free. If you smoke, give it up. If your friends and family smoke, ask them not to do it around you. Breathing in cigarette smoke takes much-needed oxygen from your body and narrows your blood vessels, making the symptoms of RP even worse.

Check out "helpful" hormones. If you take hormone replacement therapy and have developed RP, there may be a connection. A recent medical study found that women taking estrogen were much more likely to develop Raynaud's phenomenon than those who weren't taking it, or those taking estrogen plus progesterone. If you take estrogen by itself, check with your doctor to see if she might change your hormone prescription to avoid the symptoms of RP.

Condition yourself. Fight Raynaud's naturally with a technique developed by Army scientists. People in this study held their hands in a bucket of warm water while standing in the freezing cold. They did this for 10 minutes, three times a day, every other day, for a total of 18 days. At the end of the treatment, the people with Raynaud's had trained the blood vessels in their hands to stay open even when their bodies felt cold. The effects of this particular treatment lasted as long as two to three years.

Try biofeedback. This is another type of conditioning exercise in which your mind trains your body to keep the blood vessels in your hands and feet open when they should be. You can learn to "think" your fingers and toes warm. Check with your doctor to find someone who can teach you this technique.

Smooth out your stress. Stress can make RP worse even when you are not cold. Learn to relax and deal better with your stress, and your symptoms of Raynaud's phenomenon may get better, too.

Avoid the causes. Jennifer recommends making choices that won't put you in a painful situation in the first place. "Don't sit down on a cold desk in a classroom, or put your hands on a cold doorknob without something between you and the metal," she advises. "If you've been out in the cold weather and want to wash your hands when you come inside, don't use either hot or cold water — it will really hurt. Lukewarm is what you want to use."

Your best plan is to stay out of cold environments that you know will bother you, and give these natural remedies a try. Your hands and feet will thank you for it.

A challenge for the nursing mother

Nursing your baby is the most natural thing in the world. Medical science has given its stamp of approval to this process that gives your newborn all the nutrition she needs, plus antibodies to fight off infection.

But for some new mothers, nursing can signal pain and distress. If you have Raynaud's phenomenon, your nipples can suffer the same painful constriction as your fingers and toes. When this happens, you may be tempted to simply give up on nursing.

But there are some natural approaches you can take to help you through this difficult period. These could make all the difference in nursing success.

▶ Keep your entire body warm. Make sure you wear enough clothing, and nurse in a well-heated room.

▶ Apply warm compresses to help relieve nipple pain.

▶ Stay away from smoke and caffeine. These aren't good for you or your baby.

▶ Learn biofeedback. This will help you condition your blood vessels to stay open.

▶ Practice relaxation techniques. Breastfeeding can be stressful, particularly when you're having problems. By relaxing both your mind and body, you're much more likely to succeed.

An unlikely link with Raynaud's

A recent medical study uncovered a connection between Raynaud's phenomenon and H. pylori, the bacterium that can cause ulcers. A group of people who had both Raynaud's phenomenon and an H. pylori infection were given therapy for a week to get rid of the bacteria. Then they were part of a follow-up study for 12 more weeks.

Surprisingly, Raynaud's phenomenon disappeared completely in 17 percent of the people who were cured of the H. pylori infection. Even among the people who still had Raynaud's, 72 percent experienced fewer and milder attacks.

Scientists speculate that an H. pylori infection produces toxins and other substances that may affect the blood vessels. By getting rid of the bacterium, you eliminate those substances, thereby reducing attacks of Raynaud's.

However, everyone who is infected with H. pylori doesn't necessarily have Raynaud's, so scientists think other factors must be at work as well. Since the exact connection is still a mystery, you can be sure we'll see more studies on H. pylori and Raynaud's in the future.

Sinusitis

Soothe your sinuses with natural relief

What medical condition makes life tougher than even heart disease or back pain? Would you believe sinusitis? A recent study found that people who suffer from chronic sinus problems experience more pain and less pleasure in their daily activities than people with these and many other chronic medical conditions.

Your sinuses are air-filled pockets located above and behind your eyes and nose. When the mucus from your sinuses doesn't drain properly from these pockets, it builds up and can become infected. Since you can feel stuffed up at any time, how can you tell the difference between a head cold and a serious sinus condition? The U.S. Department of Health and Human Services offers this advice: When your sinus discomfort interferes with your life, causes you to miss work or take frequent naps, or is the source of regular colds, infections, or earaches, it is time to see a doctor.

One simple way to see if your sinus problem is serious is to take the jump test, a technique that Dr. Basil Rodansky, the test's inventor, swears by. Simply jump up and down or skip rope for a few minutes, and observe the results. If this causes severe sinus pain, says Rodansky, you probably have acute sinusitis and should consult your doctor.

Avoiding known irritants and allergens can help prevent mild sinus problems. When they do come up, knowing how to handle them can make your life a lot more pleasant.

Sleep soundly. Research shows that not getting enough sleep can make your sinus problems more painful and longer-lasting. Too much sleep, however, can have the same effect. Try sleeping with your head slightly raised to help your sinuses drain at night, or if one side is stuffier than the other, sleep with that side tilted down.

Run for it. For many people, mild to vigorous exercise opens up nasal passages and clears their breathing. Others find it makes their clogged sinuses worse. You should be exercising anyway, so why not give this solution a shot and see if it helps?

Care for your air. Even clean air can irritate sensitive sinuses, especially in winter months when it is particularly dry. Use a humidifier in your home to put moisture back into the air and make it easier to breathe. It will help keep your sinuses from drying out.

Go soak your head. Some people get relief by placing warm, water-soaked towels directly over their sinuses, holding their face over a steaming sink, or simply breathing in the steam from a cup of hot water. For an extra boost, consider adding pine oil, eucalyptus, or menthol to the water.

Mind your menu. Keep a careful eye on your diet, and notice if certain foods cause stuffiness. Just about anything can be a food allergen, but some common culprits are wheat, milk, and red wine.

On the other hand, some foods can actually clear your sinuses. Horseradish, garlic, and cayenne are all famous for cutting through tough sinus blocks. Mix some in with soups or other favorite foods for a quick dose of relief.

Visit the druggist. Natural solutions are best, but sometimes an over-the-counter decongestant is good for some quick relief. Try to use a decongestant that has only one active ingredient, so there will be fewer side effects, and it will be easier to stop using. Never use a decongestant for more than three days. Longer than that, and you risk developing a dependency that can cause a "rebound effect," in which the symptoms come back worse after you stop taking the medicine.

Steer clear of blockers. One type of medication you should avoid is antihistamines. These medicines basically dry up your sinuses and cause your mucus to thicken up, which may provide temporary relief but does not solve the real problem. In fact, stopping the regular flow of mucus through your sinuses can actually make the problems worse.

Rinse out your nose. It may sound uncomfortable, but many find relief through nasal rinses you can make right at home. Simply mix a quarter teaspoon of ordinary table salt with 7 ounces of warm water. With a bulb syringe, squirt the solution into your nose and let it soothe and rinse your sinuses.

You can also use a device called a Neti Pot, a spouted container designed to pour water into your nose. After mixing the salt and water in the container, tilt your head sideways over the sink and pour the solution into one nostril, letting it flow out the other, then repeat with the other nostril. After 30 seconds or so, use a tissue or your fingers to blow out whatever solution remains in your sinuses. Check your local health food store for the Neti Pot or a similar product.

Rinsing your nose daily may help you avoid colds as well as sinus problems. In a study at Pennsylvania State University, researchers showed that using a daily saline rinse significantly reduced the number of colds among college students.

Try natural relief. There are probably as many opinions out there on natural remedies as there are sinusitis sufferers.

► Some swear by acupressure, in which you apply a few seconds of direct pressure to certain sensitive spots on your face, such as the inner edges of your eyebrows, the sides of your nose, and the bones below and around your eyes.

► Light massage, especially to the area over your sinuses and the muscle between your thumb and forefinger, has been known to bring some relief.

► If all else fails, try crying. (You probably feel like it anyway.) Releasing pent-up emotion may also relieve pressure in your sinuses.

The trick is to find what works best for you, and stick with it. If home remedies fail, and you continue to get worse, make sure you see your doctor before the infection causes lasting damage.

Spicy tonics for sticky sinuses

An herbal solution might hold the cure for what ails you. Try these for some much-needed relief from your distressing symptoms.

Hot shot. Mix one-half clove of garlic with a teaspoon of cayenne, a teaspoon of honey, and the juice of one lemon. Drink this jolting mixture three times a day for a few days, and your sinuses should respond.

Spicy tea. In a cup of hot water, combine one teaspoon each of cinnamon, sage, and bay leaves with a few squirts of concentrated lemon. Drink as needed.

Chicken soup. Don't forget this old standby. A good dose of garlic, onion, and parsley in your favorite recipe will help clear your stuffy nose and make you feel better all around.

Nose 'Band-Aid' helps you breathe better

Maybe you've seen football players wearing them on TV. Or the serious jogger who runs by your house every night. Nasal strips — those little strips that look like Band-Aids across the bridge of your nose — are starting to show up all over the place, and with good reason.

These "nose springs" are designed to improve your breathing by putting slight pressure on your nasal cavity. Breathe Right nasal strips did just that in two German trials. In one study, all participants showed a significant improvement in their nasal breathing. In the other, a sleep study, the Breathe Right strips greatly reduced the amount and intensity of snoring.

Does all this mean that nasal strips can solve airflow problems based on clogged sinuses or allergies? It's possible. The small strips work like a spring to pull your nostrils open a bit. This gives you more room in your nasal passages, which makes breathing a little easier. It's certainly not a permanent solution, but it may give you the temporary relief you need. Look for them at your local drugstore.

Skin Cancer

Simple steps can save your skin

Skin cancer shows up most often in people over 50, but it begins when you are much younger. Each time you expose yourself unprotected to the sun, you raise your risk of developing skin cancer — and millions of people are doing just that every day.

The good news is that skin cancer is usually curable if diagnosed early enough. "The difference between life and death is a quarter of an inch," says Dr. Perry Robins, president of the National Skin Cancer Foundation. "If you catch it early, nobody need die." That's why the two keys to fighting skin cancer are prevention and early detection.

Begin with sun safety. The biggest enemy your skin has is the sun. Ultraviolet rays damage skin cells and can cause them to grow uncontrollably. Protecting your skin from the sun should be your number one priority.

▶ Avoid getting too much sun even during the winter and on cloudy days. Be especially careful between 10 a.m. to 3 p.m. when the sun is strongest. If you must be in the sun during this time, wear long sleeves, a hat, and sunglasses.

▶ Sunscreen is your next best defense against skin cancer. Choose a waterproof product with sun protection factor (SPF) of 15 or higher, and reapply it often.

▶ Use strong sunblock on vulnerable areas like your nose, ears, and lips. In fact, applying lipstick twice a day will cut your risk of developing lip cancer in half. Men need to remember their lips, too. There are several colorless lip balms available that contain sunscreen.

Aim for early detection. Nearly all skin cancers can be cured if found early enough. Your doctor can even remove most growths right in the office. Have her give your entire body a thorough inspection once a year, especially if you are light-skinned. Between professional exams, get in the habit of checking yourself once a month.

▶ Look at both sides of your hands and at your lower and upper arms.

▶ Undress completely and stand in front of a full-length mirror. Look at your whole body, front and back. Raise your arms so you can check under them. Use a hand mirror for any back parts you can't see.

▶ Use the hand mirror to examine your scalp, ears, and the back of your neck. Part your hair or use a blow dryer for a closer look.

▶ Check out the backs of your legs and the bottoms of your feet with the mirror. Look between your toes, too.

What you are looking for is anything new, like a change in a mole or new growths. Be on the lookout for any mole with the ABCDs listed below. They could be the deadliest form of skin cancer — malignant melanoma.

▶ **A for asymmetry.** This means that one side of a mole doesn't match the other.

▶ **B for border.** The border of most moles is smooth. A mole with edges that are irregular, ragged, or blurred could be a warning sign.

▶ **C for color.** A mole that is a mixture of colors, including blue, red, tan, black, white, or brown could be a red flag signalling melanoma.

▶ **D for diameter.** If a mole is larger than a pencil eraser, have it checked out by your doctor — it could be cancer.

Other types of skin cancer include basal and squamous cell carcinomas. They may look like a pearly bump or a red, scaly, sharply outlined patch. You may think flat moles or patches are harmless, but that's not necessarily true, so talk to your doctor about any new or different skin growths you find.

Count your way to cancer protection

Want to figure out your chances of getting skin cancer? Try counting the number of moles you have on your body. Experts say it's a fairly reliable indicator of how likely you are to develop skin cancer. By adulthood, the average person has 15 to 20 moles. If you have more than that, you have a greater risk of developing this disease.

When checking for moles, it is important to recognize the difference between these types of spots and freckles or age spots. Moles first appear as flat, dark-brown spots, but they eventually rise and become rounded, sometimes turning light brown or pink.

Liver spots or age spots are larger, flat, brown patches that usually appear after age 55, especially on the face and hands.

Warning: Sunscreen may promote skin cancer

You spend a lot of time in the sun, but you faithfully slather on sunscreen, so you don't have to worry about skin cancer, right? Think again. Researchers have now found that a major ingredient in sunscreen may actually increase your risk of developing skin cancer.

The ingredient is PBSA, and it absorbs the sun's harmful UVB waves. In laboratory tests, when PBSA was exposed to sunlight, it damaged DNA, and researchers think this type of damage within skin cells could lead to cancer. Although there's no evidence this happens in human cells, scientists believe there's enough uncertainty to justify using a different UV filter in sunscreen that doesn't attack DNA.

Although dermatologists don't want you to stop wearing sunscreen, many professionals have concerns about sunscreen and sun safety. Here are some things you should remember when shopping for sunscreen products.

Look for the right UVA protection. Some sunscreens protect you from UVB rays and sometimes the shorter UVA-II rays — but not from UVA-I. And UVA rays have been linked to sun-damaged skin. Most sunscreen labels don't tell you that. In fact, the FDA even states that the term "SPF" (sun protection factor) should not pertain to UVA protection at all.

Check the labels for ingredients that block UVA rays. They include zinc oxide, titanium dioxide, sulisobenzone, oxybenzone, benzophenone, and avobenzone (Parsol 1789). Keep in mind, though, the FDA believes no testing method can consistently measure how much UVA protection you receive from these ingredients.

Don't play by the numbers. You probably believe the higher the SPF on a product, the longer you can stay out in the sun. After, all isn't that the way the product is advertised? Experts say a major problem with SPF numbers is that they give people this false sense of security.

Yes, sunscreens do help prevent sunburn, but remember, a sunburn is your body's way of saying "enough!" Without this early warning sign, you are more likely to stay out in the sun, damaging your skin over several hours instead of minutes. That may be one reason why a study of European schoolchildren found that heavy sunscreen users have an increased risk of skin cancer.

If you're out in the sun, experts do recommend you wear a sunscreen with an SPF of at least 15, but reapply it often, especially if you're swimming. And don't rely on sunscreen alone to shield you from the sun's burning rays. By restricting your time outside and wearing protective clothing, including a hat, you'll make sure sunburn and other skin problems don't spoil your outdoor fun.

Sunny news: Vaccine may put the block on melanoma

"Slip, slap, slop." This slogan was coined to get children and adults to protect themselves from the harmful rays of the sun. Slip on a shirt, slap on a hat, and slop on sunscreen. Catchy, but is it making a difference?

Many experts don't think so. One study from the Mayo Clinic found that from 1984 to 1992, the number of cases of SCC (squamous cell carcinoma) for females more than doubled. Not good news, especially considering the increase in public awareness of skin cancer and the large number of sunscreens on the market.

But now there is hope in the form of an experimental vaccine that offers protection from melanoma, the fastest-growing, deadliest form of skin cancer. Called gm2, this vaccine uses your own immune system to destroy tumors. It must pass rigorous testing and larger patient trials before it will be approved, but for now, it has the attention — and the funding — of the National Cancer Institute.

This is good news for the future, but until this vaccine is available to the public, you'll have to rely on sunscreens and your own good judgment.

Stress

Banish stress with better breathing

In a hurry? Under pressure? Worries got you feeling low? Just slow down, relax, and take a deep breath. Simple, but good, advice.

Under stress, most people tend to breathe high up in their chests, taking short, shallow, rapid breaths. This is appropriate in times of physical danger. It's part of the "fight or flight" response you inherited from your cave-dwelling ancestors. If you need to get out of the way of a speeding car, for example, it gets you moving before you have time to think about it.

But when dealing with stresses brought on by your job or problems in your family, running away — or fighting — would only make things worse. Slower, deeper breathing can help you settle down. Once you are calm and relaxed, you can think first, then act more sensibly.

Psychologist and breathing expert Dr. Gay Hendricks is an advocate for what he calls "conscious breathing." In his book *Conscious Breathing: Breathwork for Health, Stress Release, and Personal Mastery,* he tells you how to use your breath to relieve stress, handle emotions, build energy, and improve your health.

"We can consciously take deeper, slower breaths, and we can consciously shift our breathing from chest to belly," says Hendricks. "I have seen this simple but powerful piece of information change many lives."

Breathe out negative emotions. Hendricks finds breathwork especially helpful when dealing with the "big three" emotions — fear, anger, and sadness. He says when you first feel an emotion, if you pay attention, you'll notice a change in your breathing. This awareness is your first step in dealing with what you are feeling.

And, he says, when you are ready to let go of an emotion, using your breath is the fastest way. Notice where you feel the emotion in your body. With anger, for example, you may feel stress in your jaw and neck muscles. Focus your attention on those places. And as you inhale, imagine you are breathing into the tension there. As you exhale, let yourself feel it move out of your body.

"Many times that's all it takes," says Hendricks. "I have witnessed this done a thousand times now, but it still moves me to see the look on people's faces when they learn that they are the masters of their feelings."

Bring the zest back to your life. Stress can really zap your energy. In his practice, Hendricks sees a lot of people with chronic fatigue syndrome. He helps them use their breath to regain their vitality.

"One great benefit of conscious breathing," he says, "is that it has a direct effect on energy level. Put simply, if you breathe effectively you have much more physical energy."

Research shows slow, deep breathing can be helpful not only for stress but for problems with blood pressure, asthma, or congestive heart failure. Here are some tips to help you make the most of your natural breathing ability.

- ▶ **Breathe through your nose.** Along with air, you also breathe in a lot of dust and other irritants. Your nose is designed to filter out these pollutants as well as to moisten and warm the air before it reaches your lungs. Although you may have to breathe through your mouth sometimes, your nostrils really are the best passageway.

- ▶ **Take it slow.** Men generally breathe 12 to 14 times a minute, women 14 to 15 times a minute. Experts tend to consider anything over 15 to be a signal of stress. Hendricks says with conscious breathing the rate of respiration usually slows to about 8 to 12 breaths per minute. With fewer breaths, your lungs don't have to work as much. Your heart rate will slow as well because it doesn't have to pump so hard to get oxygen through your body.

▶ **Go deep.** While most people breathe high in the chest, Hendricks recommends breathing into the belly. This doesn't mean you actually breathe air into your stomach. As you pull the air deeper into your lungs, the diaphragm drops and pushes your abdomen out as if it were filled with air. With deep breathing, the air reaches the lower area of your lungs where more blood is available to carry healthy oxygen to your organs.

▶ **Empty your lungs fully.** When you exhale, pull your abdomen in tightly to squeeze out all the old air. Then you'll have more room for plenty of fresh air on the next inhalation.

▶ **Stay in your comfort zone.** Don't push yourself to breathe so deeply or hold your breath so long that it becomes unpleasant. It should be restful, not distressing. With practice, you'll gradually get comfortable with longer, deeper breaths.

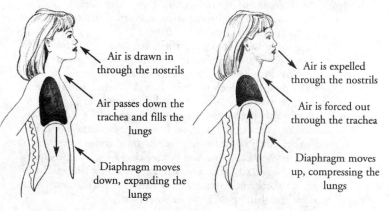

Air is drawn in through the nostrils

Air passes down the trachea and fills the lungs

Diaphragm moves down, expanding the lungs

Air is expelled through the nostrils

Air is forced out through the trachea

Diaphragm moves up, compressing the lungs

Hendricks believes that breathing will play a major role in both medicine and psychotherapy in the 21st century. Conscious breathing is within everyone's control and is easy to learn. Make it a part of your daily life, and you'll be on your way to a more relaxed, stress-free existence.

Oxygen bars may be unhealthy fad

Actor Woody Harrelson, who once played a bartender on the popular TV show "Cheers," has opened a new kind of bar in Hollywood. There, instead of ordering a shot of alcohol, you can get a "shot" of oxygen.

Bars like his are popping up in lots of big, smogged-in cities — places like New Delhi, Tokyo, and New York City. For about $1 per minute, you can hook yourself up to plastic tubes and breathe in oxygen. And if you prefer, you can have it laced with scents like orange, lemon, or mint. Promoters promise it will give you everything from more energy and sharper thinking to help with allergies, headaches, sinus problems, and even hangovers. Experts, however, aren't so sure.

First off, the Federal Food, Drug, and Cosmetic Act says any type of oxygen used for breathing and given by another person is considered a drug. Technically, these oxygen bars need a prescription to dispense oxygen, but the FDA allows each state to enforce their ruling. In addition, there are often matters of false advertising and potential health hazards.

The oxygen you get at one of these bars may claim to be as high as 99 percent pure. In fact, it's often about half that. While low levels of oxygen like this probably aren't dangerous to normally healthy people, there's no evidence at all that supplementing with oxygen will cure serious conditions and, in fact, if you have certain health problems, oxygen bars could be dangerous. The risks are real for people with asthma, emphysema, heart disease, and other lung conditions. Think, too, about the lack of regulation in oxygen bars. No one is checking to see if the equipment is cleaned regularly and working as it should. You might be inhaling oils, allergens, bacteria, or other contaminants that could lead to breathing problems or infection.

Religion: Good for the body and soul

In the old days, doctors knew that people's faith and beliefs sometimes kept them alive when medical science failed. Then, as new vaccines wiped out such devastating diseases as polio and smallpox, people began to think medical science had all the answers. The element of faith in health and healing was lost.

Now the pendulum is swinging back, and the medical profession is taking a serious look at how prayer and religious beliefs can affect their patients' health and recovery from illness. Recent scientific studies have shown some of the ways faith may work in medicine.

▶ **Helps you thrive after surgery.** In New Hampshire, doctors studied 232 older people for the critical six-month period after heart surgery. Two of the most important predictors of survival were being part of a community and having religious faith. The people who didn't have these things were much more likely to die during this time.

▶ **Heals your heart.** Another study showed that heart patients who were prayed for by a home prayer group were much less likely to need antibiotics or have complications from surgery and were less likely to die. This was true although the heart patients didn't even know they were being prayed for.

▶ **Overcomes high blood pressure.** Being a religious person can actually protect you from this serious condition. Several studies have shown that actively religious people tend to have lower blood pressure. In a North Carolina study of 112 women, spirituality proved even more important than diet, physical activity, smoking, and drinking alcohol. Researchers believe that the comfort of faith may be the key. Among other things, it improves your ability to cope with stress.

Reap the benefits of believing. Spirituality can improve overall health to such an extent that religious people actually have a lower mortality rate than people who are not religious. And you don't have to attend formal services to gain these benefits — you can be privately spiritual as well. But if you do attend and become part of a larger religious community, your health will be protected even more.

After studying more than 5,000 of the faithful for 28 years, California researchers found that religious people who get involved in their communities of faith are less likely to die from any cause. Those people who attended services most often were the healthiest of all.

Scientists think people who frequently take part in religious services may have better health practices, more social contacts, and are more likely to stay married. These are all factors that keep you in good health.

Discuss faith with your doctor. Surveys show that most people want to talk about their faith with their doctors, but most doctors have not been willing to do that in the past. This is changing as more evidence shows that faith is a factor in health and healing. Some medical schools are even adding spirituality to their courses of study. Soon more doctors should be aware of the effects religion has on the lives of their patients and be more willing to discuss it.

Put your faith to work. Knowing that your faith is a benefit to your health is a comfort in itself, but here are some active steps you can take as well.

- ▶ **Make time to pray.** Each day, dedicate time to the practice of your religious faith. Pray or meditate on your faith in whatever way is comfortable and appropriate for you. The beginning of the day is an excellent time for this private practice, but any time you can consistently set aside is fine.

- ▶ **Join a group.** A bible study or scholarly study group that meets consistently to share faith and ideas is a good source of social support. Having such friends in your life is vitally important. A recent Swedish medical study of female heart patients ages 30 to 65 showed that those without social support had a much higher risk of clogged arteries and heart attack.

- ▶ **Spend time with family and friends.** Sometimes it takes a lot of effort to get together with people you care about, but it's important for your health as well as your happiness. If you really can't get out of your home, even regular phone calls will keep the benefits of social support flowing your way.

- ▶ **Practice forgiveness and peace.** Most major religions contain an element of both these concepts. If you can let go of past hurts and feel calm about the present, you can reduce the stress in your life and all the health problems it can cause.

A sexy way to fight off stress

If someone were to ask you the question, "How often should you have sex?" you might very well answer with a smile, "As often as possible." Even though you may be joking around, the truth of the matter is — you're right!

A healthy sex life can greatly contribute to your overall health, help you feel young and energetic, and keep the spark burning bright in your relationship. It's one of life's best stress relievers and boasts a number of other benefits that can't be beat.

Battles built-up tension. Like most forms of exercise, sex is a natural stress killer. It works out and loosens up practically every muscle in your body, draining the tension that may have built up inside you over a long day. At the same time, it provides a sweet vacation for your mind, releasing your attention from the challenges in your life and refocusing, at least for a little while, on something much more pleasant.

Protects against pain. Any type of pain, particularly chronic pain, can make your life more stressful. Sex fights pain by getting you into better shape and by making you feel good in general, but it also attacks pain at a deeper level. Like most exercise, it encourages your brain to produce endorphins, chemicals that actually raise your tolerance to pain. Higher levels of endorphins in your body mean lower levels of pain in your life.

Sexual activity also challenges your muscles and joints, works out stiffness, and keeps you limber. If you have arthritis, being in good, flexible condition can help keep your symptoms under control. Flexibility is also your best protection against serious injury in case of an accident.

Improves your fitness. Excess weight can contribute to stressful feelings. And as a way to stay physically fit, amorous activity is hard to beat. Experts say that active sex burns about 300 calories. That means you could lose 12 pounds in the next year without changing your diet or working out longer. You just need to fit in some "quality time" with your spouse three or four times a week.

Dr. Susan Lark, author of *The Estrogen Decision,* says that sex helps your ovaries produce more androgens, which are the hormones that stimulate your desire. And the extra spark that brings to your relationship might be the nicest stress-beater of all.

Stroke

Watch out for hidden stroke triggers

What do snoring, drinking beer, and taking aspirin or decongestants have in common? Believe it or not, they may all give you a stroke. Knowing about such unexpected, hidden risks as these — and how to deal with them — could very well save your life.

Check your breathing. Your spouse's snoring may be so bad that you're ready to sleep in another room. But wait. Before you leave him on his own, check to make sure he's not suffering from a potentially deadly sleep disorder. Consistent snoring can be a sign of sleep apnea, a dangerous condition that could put him at severe risk for a massive stroke.

During an attack of sleep apnea, you stop breathing momentarily. The struggle to breathe causes your blood pressure to shoot up, damaging the carotid arteries that carry blood to the brain. Putting these critical arteries in jeopardy puts you at terrible risk for stroke.

Sleep apnea is seen most often in overweight people and can be treated. If you suspect you or a loved one may suffer from sleep apnea, see your doctor or visit a sleep clinic as soon as possible.

Ditch your decongestant. If you use an over-the-counter medicine to clear up that stuffy nose, you might want to reconsider. Research shows that long-term use of a common decongestant called pseudoephedrine may trigger a stroke, especially in those who suffer from migraines or Raynaud's phenomenon. If you are using this medicine and have one or more other stroke risk factors, you should ask your doctor about alternatives.

Cut your beer intake. Too much alcohol opens the door to many health problems, but heavy beer drinkers may have more to worry about when it comes to stroke risk. A study at the Innsbruck

University Clinic in Austria found that people who drink more than four beers a day tend to have more fatty buildup in the arteries leading to their brains. This type of blockage can cause an ischemic stroke. The study found that heavy beer drinking was an even bigger risk factor for stroke than smoking 20 cigarettes or more a day.

Evaluate aspirin's pros and cons. For years, you've heeded the advice to take aspirin to help control your risk of heart disease. While this may be sound advice for protecting your heart, doctors have now found it might not be so good for your brain.

Researchers at Johns Hopkins and Tulane universities analyzed 16 studies involving subjects who had suffered hemorrhagic strokes. This type of stroke occurs when a weakened artery bursts in your brain. They found that although aspirin makes you less likely to have a heart attack or ischemic stroke, it may increase your risk of having a hemorrhagic stroke.

The researchers concluded that the benefits of aspirin therapy for your heart probably outweigh the danger it poses in stroke risk. But this may not be true for all people. If you are at particular risk for hemorrhagic stroke, be sure to discuss this with your doctor before starting an aspirin-a-day routine.

Is a stroke in your future?

A blocked blood vessel in the brain or neck is the most frequent cause of stroke. It accounts for about eight out of 10 "brain attacks." Bleeding strokes, although less common, are usually more severe and more often fatal. Keep these risk factors in mind to ward off both types of stroke.

- **History of stroke.** If you have had a stroke, or if it is common in your family, you should consider yourself at a higher risk and pay close attention to other risk factors.
- **High blood pressure.** The worst risk factor of them all, hypertension increases the pressure on your arteries and makes a hemorrhage much more likely.
- **Heart disease.** An unhealthy heart that works harder and less effectively can put you in much greater danger of stroke.

- **Diabetes.** This disease may destroy blood vessels throughout your body, including your brain. If your blood sugar levels are high when you have a stroke, the damage may be more severe. Keeping your diabetes under control is the best way to prevent a stroke.
- **Unhealthy lifestyle.** Too much salt, a poor diet, smoking, and lack of exercise all help set the stage for stroke as well as for the disorders that often lead to stroke.
- **Race.** African-Americans are at a statistically higher risk. Some studies have shown that other minorities may be at an elevated risk as well.

5 ways to ward off stroke

Protecting yourself against stroke is more than just avoiding triggers that are known to cause them. By taking charge of your diet and lifestyle, you'll lower your odds of suffering a stroke even more.

Choose your fats carefully. Some fats are healthier than others, and some may even protect you against stroke. For the best defense, choose walnuts, soybean oil, and canola oil. They contain alpha-linolenic acid, which studies have found lower stroke risk. Just a handful of walnuts or a tablespoon of soybean or canola oil daily is enough to give you this important benefit.

Drink your milk. Ever heard of a cow having a stroke? Maybe it's because of the milk. Researchers have learned that the more milk you drink, the less likely you are to suffer a stroke. In fact, non-milk drinkers have double the stroke rate of people who drink at least 16 ounces every day.

Researchers aren't sure why milk has this effect since calcium from non-dairy sources does not produce the same result. It could mean that milk has an unidentified ingredient that helps prevent stroke. Or maybe the milk drinkers in the study group were just more health conscious overall. But drinking four cups a day will at least satisfy your daily calcium requirements. And it just may fortify your body against strokes as well.

Go a little bananas. A Harvard professor has "gone bananas" over the value of potassium in cutting your stroke risk. In an eight-year study published by the American Heart Association, he found that men who ate the most potassium had the lowest incidence of stroke. Like with milk and calcium, using potassium supplements won't have the same impact. You've got to eat your fruits and veggies. Try bananas, spinach, tomatoes, and oranges for a good dose of this stroke-preventing mineral.

Have a glass of wine. Studies have shown that moderate alcohol intake may reduce your risk of stroke. A new study says that if you do drink alcohol, wine should be your beverage of choice.

Dr. Thomas Truelsen of the Institute of Preventive Medicine in Copenhagen led a study that found that people who drink wine every day have 32 percent less stroke risk than people who never drink at all. The study found no such benefit for people who drink beer or liquor.

Of course, if you don't drink, you shouldn't start simply to lower your stroke risk. You can make plenty of other changes that are not as potentially harmful.

Exercise — but don't overdo it. Exercise is one of the basic building blocks of good health, but more is not always better. In fact, when it comes to stroke, exercise can only lower your risk so far, according to a Harvard report.

In a 20-year study of 11,000 men, researchers found that burning between 1,000 and 3,000 calories per week did indeed lower stroke risk. But working out harder and longer did not lower the risk any further. The study also showed that in order to be effective, exercise needed to be at least moderately strenuous — for instance, walking instead of bowling.

You can easily burn 1,000 calories by walking briskly for 30 minutes five or six times a week. Or, if you'd like some company, grab a partner for a couple of hours of doubles tennis or an evening of dancing. You'll both reap the benefits of stroke protection.

Prevent strokes with a tap of your foot

You may not be able to dance, but the National Stroke Association (NSA) wants you to at least tap your foot — so you can find out whether you're at risk of having a stroke.

Simply by measuring your heartbeat against a regular tapping of your foot, you can find out if you have atrial fibrillation (AF), a condition where your heart beats out of rhythm. This irregular heartbeat can cause blood clots that may break loose and travel to your brain — making you five times more likely to have a stroke. Atrial fibrillation is treatable, however, and by diagnosing it early, you may be able to prevent an AF-related stroke.

The National Stroke Association is excited about this self-screening technique that may help prevent some of the 80,000 strokes AF causes each year. "We are trying to raise public awareness of strokes and do everything we can to help people learn how to prevent them," says NSA's Steve Smock.

Here's how to make this toe-tapping technique work for you:

▶ Place the first two fingers of your right hand on your left wrist and find your pulse.

▶ Check your watch or clock and, for one minute, tap your foot in time to your pulse. Is your foot tapping steadily, like a clock ticking? Or is it uneven, with extra or missing beats?

If you find your foot tapping like a runaway horse, see your doctor for a more thorough screening. You should also talk to him if you have a problem finding your pulse or tapping your toes in rhythm. The technique must be done properly to give you an accurate idea of your stroke risk.

TMJ

7 ways to quit grinding your teeth

Did you know that your teeth, on average, can bite down with a force of 162 pounds per square inch (psi)? If that sounds like a lot, imagine a biting force of 975 psi — that's the record for teeth grinding. It's no wonder that this condition, called bruxism, can cause serious dental damage.

Bruxism can also lead to TMJ (temporomandibular joint disorder). The temporomandibular joints on each side of your head connect your upper and lower jaws to each other and to your skull. They allow your jaws to open and close, rotate, and move back and forth.

When these joints become damaged, it can cause pain in your ear, teeth, jaw, neck, and/or head. Some of the other symptoms of TMJ disorder are a clicking or popping sound when you open your mouth or chew, pain when you yawn, and the inability to open your mouth widely. Although there are several possible causes of TMJ, bruxism accounts for many cases.

Besides running the risk of developing TMJ, people with serious bruxism will have teeth that appear flat on the surface, because they've worn them down. You can even wear the enamel off your teeth, exposing the dentin, which is the inside part of your tooth. Your teeth then become very sensitive, particularly to temperature extremes of hot and cold.

All the painful problems bruxism can lead to makes it painfully obvious that you need to find a way to stop the grinding.

Reduce stress. The best way to eliminate teeth grinding is to get rid of the stress causing it, but for most people, stress is an inescapable fact of life. However, finding effective ways of dealing with it may help. (See the *Stress* chapter for suggestions on dealing with stress and anxiety.) Since most teeth grinding occurs at night, a relaxing bed-time ritual like taking a warm bath or reading may help. If you're under severe stress, however, counseling may be the best solution.

Change your sleeping position. The position you sleep in can make a difference. The best way to sleep is on your back with pillows or rolled-up towels under your knees and neck. This position allows your lower jaw to relax. If you can't sleep on your back, sleep on your side with supports under your head, shoulder, and arm. Sleeping on your stomach is not recommended.

Have someone wake you. Often, you don't even realize you're grinding your teeth in your sleep until your spouse complains that the noise is keeping him awake. If this is the case, ask your spouse to wake you whenever he notices you grinding away. This may help break the cycle and condition you to stop before you have to be awakened.

Get a mouthguard. Your dentist can fit you with a mouthguard, similar to the ones worn by boxers, only smaller. This device may or may not stop you from grinding your teeth, but it will at least help protect your teeth from more severe damage.

Eat soft foods. Bruxism causes your jaw muscles to become tired and overworked. Give them a break by eating soft foods and staying away from hard, chewy foods like bagels.

Avoid chewing gum. You may think chewing gum will help relieve the stress that makes you grind your teeth, but it uses those same overworked jaw muscles, so you're better off without it.

Use your imagination. Visual imagery and relaxation techniques may help reduce stress and loosen up that tight jaw. Think about relaxing your jaws with your lips closed and your teeth apart. Try to do this about 50 times a day, until you're comfortable doing it. Then visualize sleeping with your jaw in that position, and soon you may be free from the nightly grind.

Tooth and Gum Disease

12 tips for whiter, healthier teeth

Your smile is one of the first things people see. If you want to make a bright and pleasant first impression, practice good oral hygiene. Here are some tips to help you keep your teeth white and healthy.

Depend on your dentist. Periodontal disease is the most common cause of tooth loss. In fact, about 75 percent of Americans suffer from some form of this smile-stealing condition. Periodontal infection starts in your gums but can move into the tissues that hold your teeth in place and spread throughout your bloodstream. The early stages are painless. You might not know you have it until it's too late.

Regular dental checkups are critical for preventing this disease. See your dentist at least once or twice a year.

Fine tune your daily routine. Dentists no longer send you on your way with the instructions, "brush your teeth." Their new motto is, "clean your mouth." Brushing, flossing, and tongue scraping should be a basic part of your daily routine.

Get the flossing facts. Use waxed or unwaxed dental floss at least once a day to clean between your teeth. Gently move the floss up and down around each tooth. Although many people prefer flossing aids, studies show you don't need an expensive tool to floss properly.

Become a brushing expert. With so many brushes and pastes to choose from, a walk down the dental aisle in your drugstore can be a dizzying experience. If you are overwhelmed, ask your dentist for advice. Most will recommend a soft-bristled toothbrush.

Electric toothbrushes have been proven to reduce plaque, especially for people who have trouble brushing properly. Just choose a soft attachment.

Select a fluoride toothpaste that fights gingivitis as well as plaque, such as Crest Gum Care and Colgate Total. Be on the lookout for toothpastes, mouthwashes, and chewing gums containing CaviStat, a nonfluoride cavity fighter. This newly patented compound contains calcium, which restores minerals to your teeth, and arginine, an amino acid found in saliva that neutralizes bacterial acids. CaviStat is awaiting FDA approval.

Steer clear of stress. Rat studies have shown that stress increases the amount and severity of tooth decay. So relax, enjoy life, and give your teeth a break.

Chew sugar-free gum. Saliva rinses food particles from your teeth, which helps protect them from cavities. Chewing increases the amount of saliva you produce.

Slow down on sugars and starches. Choosing nutritious foods is a big part of preventing tooth decay and gum disease. Knowing what to avoid is as important as knowing what to eat. The plaque-causing bacteria in your mouth love sugars and starches. In fact, after you eat foods high in sugars or starches, these bacteria will actively attack your teeth for at least 20 minutes. You don't necessarily have to give up these foods, just clean your mouth soon after eating them. You may be surprised to learn that fruits, milk, bread, cereals, and some vegetables contain sugars or starches.

Limit between-meal snacks. When you eat a full meal, you produce a lot of saliva, which washes the bacteria and acids out of your mouth. When you eat a snack, you don't produce much saliva. That means food particles are left between your teeth. If you must snack, choose healthy ones, like fruit, raw vegetables, cheese, and yogurt, and brush your teeth afterward.

Drink lots of water. Not only will water help flush the toxins out of your body, it will rinse bacteria out of your mouth and stimulate your own production of bacteria-fighting saliva.

Sidestep these tooth stainers. Products like red wine, tea, coffee, berries, and tobacco will stain your teeth. If you can't give up your morning cup of java, remember this — coffee stains less than tea. Tea drinkers should choose light-colored herb teas because they stain less than other teas. When drinking dark liquids, use a straw. It keeps the liquid from washing over your teeth and causing stains.

Avoid acidic foods. These foods open up the pores in your tooth enamel and allow stains to discolor your teeth. To make your tea or coffee less acidic, add milk.

Be wary of drugstore bleaches. Most dentists do not recommend over-the-counter bleaching products. They think this procedure should be supervised by a professional. If you buy an OTC whitener, make sure it has the ADA Seal of Acceptance. This means it has met the American Dental Association's standards for safety and effectiveness.

How to care for sensitive teeth

If ice water makes you flinch and hot tea brings on shivers of pain, you probably have sensitive teeth. That doesn't mean the end of frozen desserts and steaming hot soups. It just means your teeth need some extra care.

- Keep brushing and flossing your teeth. This removes the bacteria that cause gingivitis and periodontal disease, two conditions that cause your gums to recede and expose the sensitive root.
- Don't brush so hard. By scrubbing with your toothbrush, you are actually brushing away gum tissue that covers and protects your tooth roots. The ALERT toothbrush has a warning light that comes on when you brush with too much pressure.
- Use a toothpaste with special ingredients for sensitive teeth. Strontium chloride causes the minerals in your saliva to harden over the pores in your exposed tooth roots, protecting the nerves inside. Potassium nitrate actually numbs the nerves in your teeth.

- Avoid high-acid foods, like citrus fruits, sodas, and tea. They open the pores in your tooth enamel and expose the nerves.
- See your dentist. He has several procedures that can help sensitive teeth.

Fast action can save that knocked-out tooth

If an accident or injury knocks out your permanent tooth, replacing it can be a traumatic, expensive procedure. Saving your natural tooth will make you and your wallet much happier. To do this, however, you must think and act quickly.

Once a tooth is knocked out of its socket, the cells on the root begin to dry up. The longer they are exposed, the less chance you have of successfully "replanting" the tooth back in your mouth. Generally, your chances of success fall by about 1 percent for every minute the tooth is out of the socket.

Dr. Tommy Turkiewicz, an Atlanta-area dentist, says time is the key to saving the tooth. "The perfect solution would be to replant the tooth within 30 minutes. But if you're within two hours, you're still going to be fine." Anything over that will require a root canal, he says.

Since timing is critical, go to your dentist first if at all possible, not the emergency room, Turkiewicz advises. Most ERs will simply put the tooth back in the socket and tell you to go see your dentist, which means you'll lose valuable time.

And just what do you do with the tooth on the way to your dentist? The best thing is to keep it in its natural environment, so try to put the tooth back into its own socket. First, hold it by the crown — never the roots — and rinse it off with water or salt water. Then gently set it back in the socket.

Turkiewicz warns that you should take extra care in replacing the tooth. "Everything is gentle here. You don't want to tear up anything as you push it back in. So gently tease it into the socket, but don't bite on it." If you can't get it back into its socket, he advises you to simply lay it inside the cheek part of your mouth.

If that doesn't work, you can also carry it in:

▶ saline solution

▶ cold milk, packed in ice

▶ commercial products from your drugstore like Hank's Balanced Salt Solution (HBSS)

These products will help preserve the tooth until you can get help.

It's tough to keep your head during a dental emergency, but knowing what to do — and doing it quickly — can make your recovery a whole lot easier.

Adapting your toothbrush for easy use

If you suffer from arthritis or some other condition that makes it hard for you to use your hands, try these tips to help make good dental hygiene a snap.

- Push the handle of your toothbrush inside a small ball made from rubber, sponge, or Styrofoam.
- Stick a sponge hair curler on the end of your toothbrush.
- Glue a bicycle grip onto your toothbrush handle.
- Lengthen the handle with a ruler, tongue depressor, or ice cream stick.
- Use an electric toothbrush.
- Use a device that holds dental floss for you.
- Attach your toothbrush to your hand using a wide rubber band, elastic bandage, or tape.
- Tie a loop in your dental floss to make it easier to grip.

Ulcers

Kill ulcer-causing bacteria with sweetness

Honey has been used for thousands of years to heal burns and wounds, but it wasn't until this century that researchers understood how the sticky stuff helped. Now they know that many varieties of honey can kill bacteria. In particular, honey made from specific flowers in New Zealand have amazing antibacterial qualities.

Active manuka honey is perhaps the most important one because it has been proven to kill *Helicobacter pylori*, the bacteria thought to cause ulcers. Researchers recommend eating the honey one hour before meals, with no fluids, and again at bedtime. Spread about one tablespoon on a piece of bread. This keeps the honey in your stomach longer, giving you maximum benefit.

You may be able to find manuka honey at a health store, but it's more likely you'll have to order it directly from the beekeepers in New Zealand. There are several distributors, so your best bet is to get hold of a computer and search the Internet to compare prices. Simply search under the term "active manuka honey," and you should come up with several ordering options.

Warts

Folksy ways to wipe out warts

The word "warts" may make you think of toads and witches, but they actually have nothing to do with either one. These pesky growths come from a virus and can appear on your hands, feet, or anywhere else the virus gets under your skin.

Warts generally are skin-colored and rough but can also be smooth, dark, and flat. They can even grow in instead of out if they're on the bottom of your foot. Those are known as plantar warts. It's important, therefore, to make sure you're dealing with a wart rather than another problem such as a corn, callus, or even a cancerous growth.

Since warts come from a virus, they will usually disappear by themselves once the virus has run its course. For this reason, many doctors will advise you to leave them alone. If you do decide to remove them by traditional means, you can expect anything from blistering skin solutions to freezing chemical treatments to laser burning.

In many cases, though, home remedies may be just as effective at clearing up the problem. Though not scientifically proven, some folks swear these solutions work just as well as medical treatments.

Take your vitamins. All you need are a few vitamin tablets and some water to mix up these wart-dissolving remedies.

- ▶ Vitamins A and E are especially good for skin problems and can be applied directly to a wart. Simply break open a capsule, squeeze the liquid on the wart, and rub it in once a day. It may take several months for the wart to disappear, so be persistent.

- ▶ Vitamin C is another effective wart fighter. Just crush up some tablets and mix with water to form a paste, and apply directly to the wart. Cover it with a bandage so the paste won't wear off. Vitamin C can irritate your skin so try to keep the mixture only on the wart.

Make these vitamins part of your regular diet to help prevent warts in the first place. Also make sure you get plenty of wart-busting nutrients like beta carotene, zinc, sulfur, and B-complex vitamins.

Check your medicine cabinet. Aspirin works just like vitamin C if you crush it and make a paste. The salicylic acid in this pain reliever will help dissolve the wart.

Play with your food. Some of the strangest-sounding wart cures come from things you eat. But they've had the most success of all, proving that folk wisdom and common sense often go hand in hand.

▶ **Bananas.** They're probably not something you think of as a medical remedy, but even some doctors swear by the banana peel treatment. Dr. Matthew Midcap, an M.D. in West Virginia, has claimed a 100-percent cure rate in treating plantar warts with bananas, even in cases where all the traditional methods had failed. Simply cut a small piece of ripe banana peel and place it over the wart, white mushy side down. Tape the peel firmly in place and wear it all day. Change the peel each day after showering. The chemicals in the peel will soften and loosen the wart, eventually killing it.

▶ **Pineapples.** While picking out your tropical fruit, don't overlook the pineapple. Pineapple juice is rich in a certain powerful enzyme that has proven an effective means of dissolving warts. Just soak a cotton ball in fresh pineapple juice, and apply it to the wart.

▶ **Potatoes.** A raw potato slice contains similar chemicals for combating warts. Rub a slice on the wart several times a day.

Turn to your garden. A final self-treatment comes from your lawn or garden (although you may not be happy to find it there.) Break open the stem of a dandelion, and apply the milky-white juice directly to the wart three times a day. After seven to 10 days, the wart should turn black and fall off.

As with any virus, successful treatment will depend on the state of your health and immune system as well as the virus itself. Don't give up if one method doesn't work for you — you can never tell what will cure your particular wart. But you may find that these folk remedies are just the thing to make your problem disappear.

Weight Control

Easy ways to boost your metabolism and burn fat

Are you a "slow burner"? One of those people who seemingly put on weight just by walking past a bakery and inhaling the aroma? If your body seems to hold onto every calorie you give it, take heart. There are ways to raise your metabolism and make your body burn those calories instead of hoarding them.

Metabolism consists of three parts: resting metabolism, which is the energy needed to maintain breathing, heart rate, and blood pressure (the number of calories burned at rest); the energy you use to digest your food; and of course, the energy required (or calories burned) while exercising.

Your resting metabolic rate (RMR) accounts for 50 to 80 percent of the calories you burn each day, so keeping it high would help you drop pounds or keep them off. Unfortunately, as you get older, your resting metabolic rate tends to slow down, which means it takes fewer calories to maintain the same weight. The problem is that most people don't eat less as they get older, and because their bodies are burning off fewer calories, weight gain is the end result.

Fortunately, research has found ways of keeping your RMR high, so you can burn more calories even while you're just watching television.

Don't crash. Crash diets may help you lose weight quickly, but they can also cause your metabolism to plummet, resulting in even quicker weight gain as soon as you fall off your diet. You can avoid this by lowering your calorie intake slowly and exercising to offset the decrease in RMR. One study found that dieting caused RMR to decrease by about 200 calories a day, but when exercise was combined with diet, RMR only decreased by 75 calories.

Muscle up your metabolism. One of the main reasons metabolism declines with age is that lean body mass also tends to decline as you get older. A pound of muscle tissue burns about 35 calories a day, but a pound of fat only uses about two calories a day. A strength-training program will not only boost your metabolism and help you lose weight, it will also make you and your bones stronger.

If you need help getting started, consult a fitness trainer or check out *Strong Women Stay Young* and *Strong Women Stay Slim* by Miriam Nelson, Ph.D. and Sarah Wernick, Ph.D. These books contain detailed advice on how to begin a strength-training program.

Get plenty of water. You may have noticed that drinking a big glass of ice water before a meal can help you feel fuller and eat less. Water can also help you make the most of your workout, so you can build more of that calorie-burning muscle.

One study found that runners who were slightly dehydrated took longer to run a race than when they drank plenty of water. So make sure you get lots of H_2O, particularly before meals and exercise.

Eat like a horse. No one would suggest you eat as much as a horse in order to raise your metabolism, but research finds that "grazing" or eating smaller, more frequent meals may boost your metabolism.

A recent study found that women over age 60 burned 30 percent less fat following a large meal of 1,000 calories than women in their 20s. However, when the women ate a smaller meal of 500 calories and then a 250-calorie snack, both age groups burned the same amount of fat.

If you divide your calories for the day into three or four light meals instead of two or three large ones, you may burn off more of what you take in.

Pick the right time to indulge. If you're a woman, you can take advantage of a certain time in your menstrual cycle to indulge in a few extra calories. Research finds that during the luteal phase (21 to 25 days after your flow starts), the amount of energy needed to absorb nutrients increases by about 20 percent.

For most women, that means they can eat about 100 extra calories a day during this time and not gain weight. Of course, if you don't eat those extra calories, you might *lose* weight.

Choose carbs over fats. Fats pack more calories than carbohydrates — 9 per gram as compared to 4 per gram. Fats also can slow down your metabolism because they're meant for long-term storage, so they burn more slowly. Carbohydrates are meant for quicker energy use, so they burn up sooner.

Eating a lot of carbohydrates can raise your RMR. One study found that vegetarians who got 62 percent of their calories from carbohydrates had RMRs that were 11 percent higher than people in the study who got only about 51 percent of their calories from carbohydrates.

So eat the right foods and stay active, and you'll keep your metabolism running high. And that's an easy way to help yourself lose weight and stay in shape.

A NEAT way to lose weight

If you drive your friends crazy by fidgeting all the time, now you have a good excuse — you're trying to lose weight.

Researchers had 16 people overeat for two months so they could measure what happened to those excess calories. Would they be stored as excess fat or burned off?

They found that the biggest factor in predicting weight gain among the overeaters was what they called the NEAT (non-exercise activity thermogenesis) factor. This was how often during the day a person changed positions, moved around, stretched, tapped their toes — in other words, fidgeted.

All the overeaters in the study gained weight, but that gain ranged from 2 pounds to 16 pounds with the more restless subjects gaining the least. Researchers speculate that the NEAT factor kicks in on some people when they overeat to compensate for the extra calories, while others just sit still and let the fat take over.

So if you've eaten a little more than you should lately, just tap your toes, drum your fingers, and fidget those extra calories away.

Quick weight loss — a quick way to gallstones

Taking off extra weight is never easy. But doctors are now saying it can actually be downright painful, especially if you're a yo-yo dieter. That's because a new study shows that people who continually take off weight and put it back on are up to 70 percent more likely to get gallstones.

Gallstones are small bits of matter — most often hardened cholesterol — that form in your gallbladder, a small organ that stores bile to help you digest fat. The stones can be extremely painful, especially if they lodge in the duct that releases bile into your intestines. Since the gallbladder is really just a storage bin, most gallstone problems are solved by your doctor removing the entire organ.

Being overweight is one of the main causes of gallstones, so taking off extra weight helps cut your risk. But it's important to lose the weight slowly and in such a way that you'll be able to keep it off. Otherwise, as the study shows, the weight loss does more harm than good.

The study followed 47,000 women for 16 years, recording their weight changes and gallstone problems. Moderate yo-yo dieters — women who went through cycles of losing 10 or more pounds only to gain it back quickly — had a 31 percent greater chance of getting gallstones than those who kept their weight steady. For severe yo-yo dieters, that number shot up to 68 percent.

Women, especially those between 20 and 60, have about twice the risk of men in developing gallstones. Pregnancy, birth control pills, and hormone replacement therapy raise your risk even more. Certain ethnic groups, such as Native Americans and Mexican-Americans, are also at higher risk.

If you are at risk for developing gallstones, particularly if you're trying to lose weight, try some preventive measures to help stop them before they start.

▶ **Bulk up with fiber.** Fiber bonds with cholesterol and helps remove it from your system, so it can't stick around and harden in your gallbladder.

▶ **Team up with water.** Water works wonders against choles-terol, too, helping to dissolve it before it has a chance to cause problems. Be sure to drink six to eight cups of water every day.

▶ **Try high C.** Some experts believe a lack of vitamin C makes you more likely to get gallstones. If you eat plenty of high-C foods like citrus fruits, you may protect yourself from gall-bladder attacks.

▶ **Don't skip meals.** Going for long periods without eating decreases gallbladder contractions. If the gallbladder doesn't contract often enough, it's more likely to form gallstones.

▶ **Avoid ultra-low-cal diets.** If you eat too little fat, the gall-bladder won't have any reason to contract and empty its bile. You need a meal or snack of about 10 grams of fat for the gall-bladder to contract normally.

Just remember, keeping your weight at a reasonable level to begin with is the best way to avoid gallstones. But if those excess pounds sneak up on you, try to lose them slowly and sensibly. If you want to begin a strict weight-loss program, discuss it with your doctor. He may decide you will benefit from ursodiol, a medication that can help prevent gallstones.

A mirror of your success

If you're serious about watching your weight, perhaps you should hang mirrors in your kitchen and dining room. Recent studies suggest that facing the image of yourself eating may help you cut out the fat.

Iowa State University psychologists Stacey Sentyrz and Brad Bushman asked college students to taste-test three kinds of cream cheese: fat-free, light, and regular. Half the students were in a room with a large mirror — the other half were in a mirrorless room. The students in the room with the mirror ate 32 percent less of the full-fat cream cheese than those who weren't forced to look at themselves as they ate.

In another study, the psychologists set up tables in a super-market for shoppers to taste full-fat, reduced-fat, and no-fat margarine spread. One table had a large mirror, and the other didn't. The shoppers at the table with the mirror ate less of the full-fat product.

So hang a mirror on the fridge, or the cookie jar, or anywhere temptation beckons. Maybe facing your worst critic will give you the incentive to make healthier choices.

5 sure-fire ways to trim your waistline

People make jokes about spare tires and bay windows. But the risk of heart disease, diabetes, and cancer is no laughing matter. The fat around your middle section raises your chances of having one of these diseases. Your buddy who carries extra pounds in other places, like maybe his hips, has a lower risk. Fortunately, there are ways to remove the excess baggage that threatens your health.

Learn to love veggies. The best way to get that string-bean shape is to eat lots of vegetables. That advice comes from scientists who followed the "expansion" of 80,000 middle-aged people for 10 years. In their study sponsored by the American Cancer Society, they found that those who ate at least 19 servings of vegetables per week were less likely to add weight at the waistline than those who ate relatively few.

If that seems like a lot of produce, try something a little different to make healthy meals more interesting. Lenore Greenstein, a dietitian from Naples, Florida, recommends foods like artichokes and hot peppers for variety when trimming down your figure.

"For those watching their waistlines, a whole artichoke is a good choice at a mere 55 calories," says Greenstein, "but that's without the butter or Hollandaise sauce. Try dipping it in some vegetable or chicken broth, mustard, or a low-fat mayonnaise."

Greenstein points out that another advantage of the artichoke is the time it takes to eat it. "It will help fill you up and control your appetite," she says.

Spicy hot jalapenos or Thai peppers are also a good choice. They contain a lot of capsaicin, which will boost your metabolism and speed up your body's ability to burn those calories.

Make the night meal a light meal. When you have a lot of food in your belly, it puts pressure on the stomach muscles, pushing them out. If you have a heavy meal and then go to bed, it's even easier for the food to put pressure on these muscles after they relax.

If you do this regularly, you'll eventually develop a potbelly. On the other hand, eating more often, but smaller amounts of food, should help flatten that tummy.

Eat, don't drink, that sweet treat. Dr. Richard Mattes, a professor of foods and nutrition at Purdue University, points out that in recent years Americans have been drinking more sweet beverages. And at the same time, our waistlines have been expanding. He's found some clues in his research as to why this may be happening.

In one experiment, when he gave people food to eat, they generally ate less at other times in the day. But this wasn't the case when he gave them something to drink. They still ate just as much later on, and since they were taking in extra calories, they gained weight.

So if you eat a dessert in the afternoon, for example, you're more likely to eat less dinner. But if your extra treat is a sugary cola or sweet lemonade, you will probably eat just as many calories as usual at mealtime. Mattes suggests you watch your total calorie intake, especially around holidays. Celebrations often call for drinking more beverages. As a result, even if you carefully avoid the buffet, you may be adding extra pounds.

If you like an extra treat between meals, you are better off choosing a solid snack. But if you really prefer a liquid treat, Mattes recommends sipping unsweetened tea, coffee or a diet drink. "By drinking a low-calorie beverage," he says, "you can enjoy the taste and sensation without adding extra calories."

Move those inches off the beltway. A group of 60- to 70-year-olds, former "couch potatoes," began jogging or walking briskly for 45 minutes four times a week. After nine to 12 months, their waistlines were an inch to an inch and a half trimmer. And researchers said it was fat, not fat-free mass, that they lost.

So if you find yourself sitting around watching your middle expand, it's time to get up and get active. And while you are at it, suck in that belly, especially when running. It may not be easy to do, but letting your stomach bounce up and down weakens your abdominal muscles. This is especially true if you slouch as you run.

Also, don't forget to stretch your hamstrings after you run. Tightening these muscles on the backs of your thighs will help you avoid a swayback that can make a potbelly more obvious.

Exercise your power to pull in the paunch. Some experts recommend weight-bearing exercises — like modified push-ups — 30 minutes per day, three or four times a week. They believe this type of exercise will help you lose more of the fat that forms in those extra inches around the middle.

Other exercises will improve your posture and help keep your stomach from sticking out. Sit-ups strengthen the upper abdominals, and pelvic tilts do the same for the lower abs. And any exercise that strengthens your lower back will help you hold your stomach in.

With these good habits, you can reduce that paunch. And then you won't be mistaken for a laughing Buddah — just a happy Joe (or Josephine), smiling all the way to a longer, healthier life.

Pick peas for low-fat protein

Did you know that a cup of green peas has more protein than a large egg? And that's without the fat and cholesterol.

Florida dietitian Lenore Greenstein suggests you eat nutritious peas year round. Fresh ones, she says, are good eaten raw in salads or stir fried. Select the "petite" variety to have on hand in the freezer.

And she says, "Dried split peas, which keep for many months, can be used for wonderful soups and stews and are a great vegetarian alternative to meats and other animal protein."

Getting more of your protein from plant sources is a good idea. A study by the American Cancer Society found that people who ate more than three servings of meat a week added extra fat around their mid-section. This increases the risk of heart disease, diabetes, and some cancers.

Fruit juice — a dieter's secret weapon

Looking for a delicious, safe way to cut a few extra calories out of your diet? Try drinking a cold, refreshing glass of orange juice or other fruit juice before meals.

According to a Yale study, drinking a glass of fructose-rich fruit juice a half-hour to an hour before a meal may help you eat less and still feel full. The study gave overweight people either an aspartame-sweetened diet drink, a glucose-water solution, a fructose-water solution, or plain water before lunch. Fructose is the type of sugar that is found in fruits.

The men who drank the fructose drink ate nearly 300 fewer calories at lunch, and the women who drank the fructose drink ate an average of 431 fewer calories, compared to people who drank plain water.

The drink itself contained about 200 calories, which means each person saved between 100 to 231 calories. At three meals a day, that could save you at least 2,100 calories a week!

If you stirred a little pectin into your orange juice, you might be able to cut out even more calories. Pectin is a complex carbohydrate, made from certain ripe fruit, which is used to thicken jams and jellies.

One study found that people who drank a glass of orange juice with a small amount of pectin added felt fuller and ate less. Other studies have found that pectin can favorably affect blood sugar levels and cholesterol.

If you've resorted to over-the-counter or prescription appetite suppressants to control your eating habits, it's nice to know that an occasional glass of tasty fruit juice before meals could be a healthy alternative.

Power up your diet

One way to get more nutritional punch from foods is to pack them with powerful vitamins and other nutrients. Today, scientists are doing just that so you can get even more nutritional value for your dollar.

For example, researchers at the University of Nevada have grown a plant whose seeds yield eight times more vitamin E than normal plant seeds. If this process can be repeated in other seed oil plants, like corn, soy, and canola, we may soon have much richer sources of one of our most essential vitamins.

Texas A&M University's Vegetable Improvement Center has created a sweeter carrot containing more beta carotene, a nutrient that converts to vitamin A in your body. And according to the Department of Agriculture, super tomatoes packed with 10 to 25 times more beta carotene will soon be available in your supermarket produce section.

Another nutrient, called inulin, is found in such foods as garlic, chicory root, leeks, and Jerusalem artichokes. Researchers say that fortifying foods with inulin will help us reap the beneficial effects of this powerful carbohydrate. These include fighting off colon cancer and preventing digestive problems such as constipation and colitis.

Chances are, you're going to see more and more of these "functional foods." By taking advantage of these super-fortified fruits and vegetables, you can be sure you're getting a nutritious, well-balanced diet.

Sources

Acne

Acne, American Academy of Dermatology <http://www.aad.org> retrieved March 12, 1999

Alternative Medicine (23,414:22)

British Medical Journal (316,7133:723)

Fix It, Clean It, and Make It Last: The Ultimate Guide to Making Your Household Items Last Forever, FC&A Publishing, Peachtree City, Ga., 1998

Medical Journal of Australia (153,8:455)

Natural Medicines and Cures Your Doctor Never Tells You About, FC&A Publishing, Peachtree City, Ga., 1995

Nursing99 Drug Handbook, Springhouse Corporation, Springhouse, Penn., 1999

U.S. Pharmacist (21,4:66)

Allergies

Allergic Rhinitis <http://www.pharm.sunysb.edu/classes/hbh330-331/MorrisLecture/Allergy/AllergicRhinitis.htm> retrieved March 15, 1999

Allergy Proceedings (12,2:113)

Annals of Allergy (63,6[Part 1]:477)

Antihistamine Class Monograph, Healthtouch Drug Information <www.healthtouch.com> retrieved March 19, 1999

How to Cool Hay Fever, The Physician and Sportsmedicine <http://www.physsportsmed.com/issues/1997/07jul/hay.htm> retrieved March 15, 1999

Jonathan Bernstein, M.D., Assistant Professor of Allergy and Immunology, University of Cincinnati School of Medicine

Journal of Allergy and Clinical Immunology (86,6[Part 1]:954)

Survive Ragweed by Limiting Exposure <http://www.allergyasthma.com/archives/allergy06.html> retrieved March 15, 1999

Vaccination Can Prevent Allergy Symptoms, Public Communications, Inc. <http://www.newswise.com/articles/VACCINAT.PCI.html> retrieved Dec. 11, 1998

Your Body's Many Cries for Water, Global Health Solutions, Inc., Falls Church, Va., 1997

Alzheimer's Disease

American Journal of Epidemiology (141,11:1059 and 142,5:515)

Annals of Neurology (36,1:100)

Possible New Risk Factor for Alzheimer's Disease, Alzheimer's Association <www.alz.org/news/rtriskfactor.htm> retrieved March 11, 1999

Science (265,5177:1464)

Angina

Angiogenesis May Be Stimulated By EECP Therapy, EECP.com news <http://www.eecp.com/news/release_1198.htm> retrieved March 16, 1999

Archives of Family Medicine (6,3:296)

Arthritis Today (13,1:58)

Facts About Angina, National Heart, Lung, and Blood Institute, <http://www.nhlbi.nih.gov/cardio/other/gp/angina.htm> retrieved March 18, 1999

Geriatric Nursing (17,2:60)

Medical Tribune, Internist and Cardiologist Edition (37,11:6)

Money (27,4:114)

Pharmacy Times (63,3:30)

Psychology Today (31,6:16)

The Journal of the American Medical Association (275,15:1143 and 279,15:1200)

Time (52,21:93)

U.S. Pharmacist (24,2:1999)

Unstable Angina, Medscape <http://www.medscape.com/govmt/AHCPR/patient/UnstableAngina.html> retrieved March 16, 1999

USA Today (Dec. 8, 1998, 10D)

Arthritis

American Family Physician (55,1:22)

Annals of Internal Medicine (125,5:353)

Annals of the Rheumatic Diseases (56,7:432)

Archives of Internal Medicine (156,18:2073)

Arthritis and Rheumatism (39,4:648 and 41,1:81)

Arthritis Today (10,1:12,22; 10,3:34; 11,3:41; 12,5:46; 13,1:12,21; and 13,3:6)

Clinical Pharmacology and Therapeutics (63,5:580)

Dr. Paul Lam, Sydney, Australia

Epidemiology (7,3:256)

Fitoterapia (68,6:483)

Geriatrics (51,11:63 and 53,2:84)

Herbal Medicine, Beaconsfield Publishers Ltd., Beaconsfield, England, 1991

Infectious Medicine (14,8:637)

Journal of the American College of Nutrition (13,4:351)

King's American Dispensatory, Eclectic Medical Publications, Sandy, Ore., 1993

Medical Update (20,6:4)

Molecular and Cellular Biochemistry (169,1:125)

MSM Methylsulfonylmethane Facts Page
<http://www.worldimage.com/products/msm/msmfacts.html> retrieved March 19, 1999

Natural Way (4,6:34)

Postgraduate Medicine (93,1:89)

Salmonella, USDA Bad Bug Book
<http://vm.cfsan.fda.gov/~mow/chap1.html> retrieved April 1, 1999

Salmonella Enteritidis Infection, Centers for Disease Control
<http://www.cdc.gov/ncidod/publications/brochures/salmon.htm>
retrieved April 1, 1999

Tai Chi for Arthritis, Arthritis Victoria <www.arthritisvic.org.au/management/exercise/taichi.htm#trained> retrieved Jan. 7, 1999

The American Journal of Clinical Nutrition (67,1:129)

The Honest Herbal, The Haworth Press, Binghamton, N.Y., 1993

U.S. Pharmacist (18,8:20 and 23,8:66)

Asthma

Archives of Physical Medicine and Rehabilitation (73,8:717)

Biochemical Pharmacology (54,7:819)

Conscious Breathing: Breathwork for Health, Stress Release, and Personal Mastery, Bantam Books, New York, 1995

Environmental Nutrition (18,12:3)

Hamilton and Whitney's Nutrition Concepts and Controversies, West Publishing Company, St. Paul, Minn., 1994

Herbal Medicine, Beaconsfield Publishers Ltd., Beaconsfield, England, 1988

Herbs of Choice: The Therapeutic Use of Phytomedicinals, The Haworth Press, Binghamton, N.Y., 1994

Journal of Asthma (35,8:667)

Natural Medicines and Cures Your Doctor Never Tells You About, FC&A Publishing, Peachtree City, Ga., 1998

Pharmacy Times (62,1:77)

Pneumologie (48,7:484)

Recommended Dietary Allowances, National Academy Press, Washington, 1989

Super LifeSpan, Super Health, FC&A Publishing, Peachtree City, Ga., 1997

The Honest Herbal, The Haworth Press, Binghamton, N.Y., 1994

The Lawrence Review of Natural Products, Facts and Comparisons, St. Louis, Mo., 1994

The Nutrition Desk Reference, Keats Publishing, New Canaan, Conn., 1995

The PDR Family Guide to Nutrition and Health, Medical Economics Co., Montvale, N.J., 1995

USDA Nutrient Values <http://www.rahul.net/cgi-bin/fatfree/usda/usda.cgi> retrieved Nov. 24, 1997

Athlete's Foot

Athlete's Foot <http://www.aad.org/aadpamphrework/AthletFoot.html> retrieved March 15, 1999

Emergency Medicine (28,11:25)

Back Pain

American Family Physician (52,5:1341,1347)

Back in Shape: Prevention and Treatment of Back Pain, Tennessee Medical Association <www.medwire.org> retrieved March 22, 1999

Back Pain, Medical Information Series, Arthritis Foundation, P.O. Box 19000, Atlanta, Ga. 30326

Medical Update (14,10:4)

Natural Medicines and Cures Your Doctor Never Tells You About, FC&A Publishing, Peachtree City, Ga., 1996

Oh My Aching Back — What You Should Know About Preventing and Treating Low Back Pain, The Journal of the American Medical Association Patient Page <www.ama-assn.org> retrieved March 22, 1999

The Health Answer Book: The Complete Guide to Symptoms, Causes, and Natural Cures for Hundreds of Health Problems, FC&A Publishing, Peachtree City, Ga., 1997

Bad Breath

Environmental Nutrition (19,12:3)

Health News (13,6:4)

Natural Health, MDX Health Digest (24,2:56,58)

Nature's Prescriptions: Foods, Vitamins, and Supplements That Prevent Disease, FC&A Publishing, Peachtree City, Ga., 1998

The Atlanta Journal/Constitution (Feb. 4, 1999, F9)

The Health Answer Book: The Complete Guide to Symptoms, Causes, and Natural Cures for Hundreds of Health Problems, FC&A Publishing, Peachtree City, Ga., 1997

Bladder Infections

Answers to Your Questions About Urinary Tract Infections, American Foundation for Urologic Disease, 1993

Science News (151,17:255)

The Health Answer Book: The Complete Guide to Symptoms, Causes, and Natural Cures for Hundreds of Health Problems, FC&A Publishing, Peachtree City, Ga., 1997

The Journal of the American Medical Association (271,10:751)

The Lawrence Review of Natural Products, Facts and Comparisons, St. Louis, Mo., 1994

The New England Journal of Medicine (339, 10:700)

Urinary Tract Infection, Nidus Information Systems, Inc., New York, 1998

Breast Cancer

American Institute for Cancer Research Newsletter (No. 59)

American Journal of Epidemiology (147,4:333)

Archives of Internal Medicine (158,1:41)

British Journal of Cancer (73,5:687)

Cancer Epidemiology, Biomarkers and Prevention (6,11:887)

Cherry Hamburgers Lower in Suspected Carcinogens, Newswise <http://www.newswise.com/articles/1998/12CHRYBURG.ACS.html> retrieved April 23, 1999

Journal of the National Cancer Institute (88,6:340 and 90,22:1724)

National Cancer Institute <http://www.nci.nih.gov> retrieved Sept. 10, 1998

The Journal of the American Medical Association (278,17:1407 and 279,7:535)

What You Need to Know About Breast Cancer, National Institutes of Health Publication No. 93-1556

Burns

American Academy of Dermatology news release (March 20, 1999)

Burn Facts, Nortrade Medical, Inc. <http://www.burnfree.com> retrieved May 11, 1999

Environmental Nutrition (21,2:8)

Kitchen Wise, Honolulu Fire Department <http://www.htdc.org> retrieved May 11, 1999

Natural Medicines and Cures Your Doctor Never Tells You About, FC&A Publishing, Peachtree City, Ga., 1998

Pharmacy Times (64,5:53)

Scott M. Dinehart, M.D., Associate Professor of Dermatology, University of Arkansas

Carpal Tunnel Syndrome

Arthritis Today (11,3:9)

British Medical Journal (316,7133:731)

Consumer Reports on Health (10,2:8)

Current Medical Diagnosis and Treatment, Appleton & Lange, Stamford, Conn., 1997

Exercises May Prevent Carpal Tunnel Syndrome, American Academy of Orthopaedic Surgeons <http://www.aaos.org> retrieved March 15, 1999

Preventing Wrist Pain and Strain, Dreyfuss Hunt, Inc., P.O. Box 35280, Boston, MA 02135

Sitting Posture: The Overlooked Factor in Carpal Tunnel Syndrome, Dennis Zacharkow, P.T. <http://www.zackback.com> retrieved March 15, 1999

The American Medical Association Encyclopedia of Medicine, Random House, New York, 1989

The Journal of the American Medical Association (280,18:1601)

The Lancet (351,9095:41)

The Physician and Sportsmedicine (26,5:15)

Cataracts

Annals of Epidemiology (6,1:41))

Cataract Information for Patients, National Eye Institute <http://www.nei.gov> retrieved Feb. 19, 1999

Cataracts Don't Respect Age, Third Age News <http://www.thirdage.com> retrieved Dec. 10, 1998

EyeNet, American Academy of Ophthalmology <http://www.eyenet.org> retrieved Feb. 15, 1999

Nature's Prescriptions: Foods, Vitamins, and Supplements That Prevent Disease, FC&A Publishing, Peachtree City, Ga., 1998

Ophthalmology (105,5:831 and 105,9:1751)

The American Journal of Clinical Nutrition (64,5:761 and 66,4:911)

The Journal of the American Medical Association (280,8:714)

Cervical Cancer

Cancer Epidemiology, Biomarkers and Prevention (1,2:119)

Cervical Cancer, The American Cancer Society <http://www3.cancer.org> retrieved April 1, 1999

Cervical Cancer, The National Women's Health Information Center <http://www.4women.org> retrieved March 29, 1999

Folic Acid, The National Women's Health Information Center <http://www.4woman.gov> retrieved March 29, 1999

USDA Nutrient Database <http://www.rahul.net/cgi-bin/fatfree/usda> retrieved April 1, 1999

Cholesterol

American Druggist (215,2:22)

FDA Talk Paper (May 20, 1998)

Healthy Heart Handbook: Control Your Cholesterol, Lower Your Blood Pressure, and Clean Your Arteries — Naturally, FC&A Publishing, Peachtree City, Ga., 1999

Hippocrates (12,7:14)

Ketchup: Good for hamburgers and your health <http://www.post-gazette.com:80/businessnews/19981217ketchup2.asp> retrieved Dec. 17, 1998

Lipids (33,10:981)

Medical Sciences Bulletin (Issue 244)

Perilla: Botany, Uses and Genetic Resources, David M. Brenner <http://newcrop.hort.purdue.edu/newcrop/proceedings1993/V2-322.html> retrieved March 2, 1999

The Atlanta Journal/Constitution (June 18, 1998, G3)

The Journal of the American Medical Association (272,17:1335)

The Lawrence Review of Natural Products, Facts and Comparisons, St. Louis, Mo.

Chronic Pain

American Journal of Medical Science ((298,6:390)

Archives of Physical Medicine and Rehabilitation (78,11:1200)

Arthritis Today (12,4:48 and 12,6:27)

Eccentrics, Dr. David Weeks <http://www.authorsspeak.com/weeks_0196.html> retrieved April 13, 1999

Laughter research conducted at LLUMC, Loma Linda University & Medical Center <http://www.llu.edu/news/today/mar99/sm.htm> retrieved April 13, 1999

Prolo Your Pain Away! Curing Chronic Pain with Prolotherapy, Beulah Land Press, Oak Park, Ill., 1998

Prolotherapy <www.caringmedical.com> retrieved March 24, 1999

The Atlanta Journal/Constitution (April 17, 1999, E3)

What is Prolotherapy? <http://www.prolotherapy.com> retrieved March 24, 1999

Colds and Flu

Alternative Medicine: The Definitive Guide, Future Medicine Publishing, Inc., Puyallup, Wash., 1993

Centers for Disease Control and Prevention <http://www.cdc.gov> retrieved Feb. 12, 1999

FDA Consumer (30,8:15)

Hippocrates (12,11:26)

Journal of Alternative and Complementary Medicine (1,4:361)

PDR for Herbal Medicines, Medical Economics Company, Inc., Montvale, N.J., 1998

Pharmacy Times (64,10:62)

Preliminary Study Proves Centuries of Herbalists Right About Echinacea, University of Florida's Institute of Food and Agricultural Sciences

Educational Media & Services news release <http://www.ifas.ufl.edu/~newsifas/99_0303.html> retrieved April 7, 1999

The Journal of the American Medical Association (277,24:1940 and 279,24:1999)

The Lawrence Review of Natural Products, Facts and Comparisons, St. Louis, Mo.

Tyler's Herbs of Choice: The Therapeutic Use of Phytomedicinals, The Haworth Press, Inc., Binghamton, N.Y., 1999

Colon Cancer

A Clove of Garlic a Day May Keep Cancer Away, MSNBC <http://www.msnbc.com> retrieved April 14, 1999

American Family Physician (59,2:261)

American Journal of Epidemiology (148,8:761)

Annals of Internal Medicine (128,9:713 and 129,7:517)

Anticancer Drugs (8,5:470)

Anticancer Research (16,5A:2911)

Biomedical and Environmental Sciences (11,3:258)

British Journal of Cancer (76,5:678 and 79,7-8:1283)

Calcium Supplements May Reduce Colon Cancer Risk, University of Iowa College of Medicine <http://www.newswise.com> retrieved Jan. 18, 1999

Cancer (80,5:858)

Cancer Epidemiology Biomarkers and Prevention (6,9:677 and 6,10:769)

Cancer Letters (95,1-2:221)

Carcinogenesis (19,8:1357)

Chopping and Cooking Affect Garlic's Anti-Cancer Activity, Penn State <http://www.psu.edu> retrieved March 18, 1999

Code of Federal Regulations: 21 CFR 101.76

Consumer Reports on Health (10,9:6)

Emergency Medicine (31,2:93)

Epidemiology (9,4:385)

Food and Chemical Toxicology (36,9:761)

General Vegetarian Diet Information For All Ages, The American Dietetic Association <http://www.healthtouch.com>

Geriatrics (51,12:45)

Hunan I Ko Ta Hsueh Hseuh Pao (22,3:246)

Journal of Cancer Research and Clinical Oncology (118,6:447)

Journal of Cellular Biochemistry (27S:100)

Journal of Investigative Dermatology (111,4:656)

Journal of Laboratory and Clinical Medicine (130,6:576)

Nutrition and Cancer (29,2:152 and 30,2:85,163)

Pharmaceutical Research (9,12:1668)

Proceedings of the National Academy of Sciences (95,19:11301)

The Atlanta Journal/Constitution (Sept. 15, 1998, F1)

The New England Journal of Medicine (340,3:169)

Vegetarian Diet Pyramid, Cornell University
<http://www.news.cornell.edu> retrieved March 29, 1999

Constipation

Clinician Reviews (8,4:130)

Gut (38,1:28)

Health News (3,13:4)

Journal of the Royal Society of Medicine (87,1:9)

The American Journal of Clinical Nutrition (62,6:1212)

Depression

Acta Neurologica Scandinavica Supplementum (154:7)

American Health (16,5:26)

American Journal of Medicine (83,5A:81,89)

Archives of Family Medicine (5,5:259 and 6,5:445)

Archives of General Psychiatry (55:161)

Archives of Internal Medicine (156,5:521)

Blood Purification (7,1:39)

British Medical Journal (313,7052:253)

Health Psychology (14,4:341)

Journal of Psychiatric Research (24,2:177)

National Vital Statistics Report (47:4)

Newsweek (133,12:65)

Psychiatry Research (56,3:295)

Psychotherapy and Psychosomatics (59,1:34)

The American Journal of Clinical Nutrition (62,1:1)

The Lancet (351,9110:1213)

The Physician and Sportsmedicine (23,9:44)

Tufts University Health & Nutrition Letter (14,12:8)

Virus may promote mood disorders, Mental Health Net & CMHC Systems <http://www.cmhc.com> retrieved May 27, 1999

Your Health (37,8:26)

Diabetes

A Podiatrist's Experience with Collagen, The Wound Care Institute, Inc. <http://woundcare.org/newsvol1n2/n2za.htm> retrieved March 9, 1999

American Journal of Pain Management (9,1:8)

Annals of Internal Medicine (130,2:89)

Biochemical and Biophysical Research Communications (244,3:678)

Diabetes Care (20,4:537 and 21:1266)

Diabetes Facts and Figures, American Diabetes Association <www.diabetes.org/ada/c20f.asp> retrieved March 22, 1999

Diabetes Info, American Diabetes Association <www.diabetes.org/ada/c20a.asp> retrieved March 12, 1999

Geriatrics (51,11:19)

Journal of the American College of Nutrition (17,6:595)

Louise Peck, Assistant Professor, Department of Foods, Science and Human Nutrition, Washington State University

Nature's Prescriptions: Foods, Vitamins, and Supplements That Prevent Disease, FC&A Publishing, Peachtree City, Ga., 1998

Nutrition Recommendations and Principles for People With Diabetes Mellitus, American Diabetic Association <www.diabetes.org> retrieved March 23, 1999

Sean Ison, Pedorthist, McMahon Shoes, Dunwoody, Ga.

The Journal of the American Medical Association (277,6:472 and 280,2:202)

What is Diabetes? <http://diabetes.com/L3TABLES/L3T100117.htm> retrieved March 11, 1999

Diverticulosis

British Journal of Surgery (78,2:190)

Diverticulosis and Diverticulitis, NIH Publication No. 97-1163, National Digestive Diseases Information Clearinghouse, 2 Information Way, Bethesda, MD 20892-3570

Hamilton and Whitney's Nutrition Concepts and Controversies, West Publishing Company, St. Paul, Minn., 1994

The Medical Advisor: The Complete Guide to Alternative and Conventional Treatments, Time-Life Books, Alexandria, Va., 1996

Drug Reactions

Archives of Internal Medicine (158,20:2200)

British Medical Journal (313,7072:1624)

Herbs for Health (3,5:34,39)

Hippocrates (12,6:46)

The Journal of the American Medical Association (271,20:1609)

Time (152,21:58)

U.S. Pharmacist (23,5:80)

Dry Eyes

Archives of Ophthalmology (115,1:34)

Dry Eye in Sjogren's Syndrome, J. Daniel Nelson, M.D., FACS <www.sjogrens.org/eye.htm> retrieved March 30, 1999

Pharmacy Times (63,12:41 and 62,4:40)

U.S. Pharmacist (23,1:38)

What's the best way to put in eye drops? Health Centre Online
<www.pharmasave.com/faq.eyedrops.htm> retrieved Feb. 11, 1999

Dry Mouth

New York Times, MDX Health Digest (138,47:965)

Oral Care for Patients with Sjogren's Syndrome, National Sjogren's
Syndrome Association <http://www.sjogrens.org/oral.htm> retrieved
March 30, 1999

*The Health Answer Book: The Complete Guide to Symptoms, Causes, and
Natural Cures for Hundreds of Health Problems*, FC&A Publishing,
Peachtree City, Ga., 1997

What is Sjogren's Syndrome <http://www.sjogrens.com/whatis.htm>
retrieved March 30, 1999

Dry Skin

Acta Dermato-Venereologica (72,5:327 and 71,1:79)

Archives of Dermatology (134,11:1401)

Dermatology (194,3:247)

Healthline (13,11:6)

Herbs of Choice: The Therapeutic Use of Phytomedicinals, The Haworth
Press, Inc., Binghamton, N.Y., 1994

Procter & Gamble news release (March 22, 1999)

Enlarged Prostate

Archives of Internal Medicine (158,21:2349)

The Journal of the American Medical Association (280,18:1604)

Eyestrain

Computer RX, Eye Clinic of Fairbanks
<www.eyeclinicfbks.com/ComputerGlasses.htm> retrieved Feb. 22, 1999

Dr. Richard Lee, Ophthalmologist, Oakland, Calif.

Kathleen Largo, Researcher, Peachtree City, Ga.

Falling

Don't let a fall be your last trip, American Academy of Orthopaedic
Surgeons <http://www.aaos.org> retrieved March 12, 1999

Journal of Psychosomatic Research (33,2:197)

Journal of the American Geriatric Society (41,3:329)

The Journal of the American Medical Association (273,17:1341)

Journals of Gerontology. Series B, Psychosocial Sciences and Social Sciences
(52,5:242)

Karen Sifton, Tai chi instructor, State University of West Georgia,
Carrollton, Ga.

Mike Ellis, Tai chi student, State University of West Georgia, Carrollton,
Ga.

Precautions can prevent falls in the home, Medscape
<http://www.medscape.com> retrieved March 16, 1999

The New England Journal of Medicine (339,13:875)

Fibromyalgia

Dottie Abbott, Tai chi student, Carrollton, Ga.

Fibromyalgia Basics, Fibromyalgia Network <www.fmnetnews.com>
retrieved Jan. 14, 1999

Rita Evans, LCSW, CCM, DeKalb Medical Center, Decatur, Ga.

U.S. Pharmacist (22,12:41)

Foot Pain

The Health Answer Book: The Complete Guide to Symptoms, Causes, and Natural Cures for Hundreds of Health Problems, FC&A Publishing, Peachtree City, Ga., 1997

The Associated Press (October 1994)

The Physician and Sportsmedicine (25,2:6 and 26,2:24)

Medical Tribune (38,6:32)

Alternative Medicine Digest (22:24)

Forgetfulness

Encyclopedia of Nutritional Supplements, Prima Publishing, Rocklin, Calif., 1996

Environmental Nutrition (21,10:1)

Journal of the American Geriatric Society (46,10:1199 and 46,11:1407)

Natural Medicines and Cures Your Doctor Never Tells You About, FC&A Publishing, Peachtree City, Ga., 1998

Natural Way (4,6:69)

Nature's Prescriptions: Foods, Vitamins, and Supplements That Prevent Disease, FC&A Publishing, Peachtree City, Ga., 1998

Neurology (41,5:644)

Neuroscientists Tie Stress to Memory Lapses, University of California, Irvine <http://www.newswise.com> retrieved March 11, 1999

Super LifeSpan, Super Health, FC&A Publishing, Peachtree City, Ga., 1997

Vitamin Deficiency May Cause Memory Problems, Net Health <http://www.alzhheimers.com> retrieved April 5, 1999

Gout

Advances in Experimental Medicine and Biology (431:839)

American Family Physician (59,4:925)

FDA Consumer (29,2:19)

Fleischerei (43,12:1122)

Hamilton & Whitney's Nutrition Concepts and Controversies, West Publishing Company, St. Paul, Minn., 1994

Nippon Rinsho (54,12:3369)

Therapeutische Umschau (52,8:524)

Hair Loss

American Family Physician (51,6:1527)

Archives of Dermatology (134,11:1349)

Dr. Amy McMichael, Dermatologist, Wake Forest University

Hair Today, Gone Tomorrow: Early Diagnosis is the Key to Treating Hair Loss in Women, American Academy of Dermatology news release, March 21, 1999

Into Thin Hair, American Academy of Dermatology <www.aad.org> retrieved March 15, 1999

Postgraduate Medicine (85,6:53)

Headaches

American Family Physician (47,4:799)

British Medical Journal (314,7091:1364)

Cephalalgia (16,4:257 and 18,10:704)

Clinical Psychiatry News (26,11:9)

Consumer Reports on Health (5,7:72)

Diet and Headache, National Headache Foundation <www.headaches.org> retrieved Aug. 15, 1997

Headache (34,10:590)

Headache Quarterly (9:159)

Headache — Guide to Treatments, Mayo Clinic Health Oasis
<www.mayohealth.org> retrieved March 31, 1999

Headache, Mayo Health Oasis <www.healthnet.ivi.com> retrieved July
21, 1997

Impurities confirmed in dietary supplement 5-hydroxy-L-tryptophan, FDA
Talk Paper, Food and Drug Administration, Aug. 31, 1998

International Archives of Allergy and Immunology (110,1:7)

Message for Users of 5-HTP, Mayo Clinic
<http://www.mayo.edu/news/5HTP/Users.html> retrieved April 8, 1999

*Nature's Prescriptions: Foods, Vitamins, and Supplements That Prevent
Disease*, FC&A Publishing, Peachtree City, Ga., 1998

Nutrition Research Newsletter (14,2:25; 15,10:109; and 15,11/12:122)

The Lancet (2,8604:189)

The Lawrence Review of Natural Products, Facts and Comparisons, St.
Louis, Mo., 1994

The National Headache Foundation, 5252 N. Western Ave., Chicago, IL
60625

Hearing Loss

American Family Physician (46,3:851; 47,5:1219; and 48,2:254)

Earwax, The Natural Remedies Encyclopedia
<http://www.pathlights.com/nr_encyclopedia> retrieved March 26, 1999

Emergency Medicine (24,15:165)

Geriatrics (53,8:69)

Hamilton and Whitney's Nutrition Concepts and Controversies, West
Publishing Co., St. Paul, Minn., 1994

Journal of Gerontological Nursing (19,4:23)

Journal of Longevity (4,5:31)

Medical Tribune for the Family Physician (34,22:2)

Postgraduate Medicine (91,8:58)

The American Journal of Clinical Nutrition (69,3:564)

The Journal of Nutrition (120,7:726)

The Lancet (351,9113:1411 and 352,9136:1240)

U.S. Pharmacist (18,4:101 and 18,12:26)

Heart Disease

American Heart Journal (134,5:974)

American Journal of Cardiology (77,14:1230)

American Journal of Epidemiology (148,5:445)

American Journal of Physiology (275,[2]:R1468)

Arteriosclerosis, Thrombosis, and Vascular Biology: Journal of the American Heart Association (18,12:1902)

British Medical Journal (317,7161:775 and 317,7167:1253)

Cardiology Clinics (14,2:263)

Chest (114,6:1556)

Circulation (97:1461)

Dean Hutsell, Meteorologist, National Weather Service

Dr. Dean Ornish's Program for Reversing Heart Disease, Random House, N.Y., 1990

Estrogen boosts risk in women with heart disease <dailynews.yahoo.com> retrieved March 17, 1999

European Heart Journal (19SC:C12)

Exercising Just Three Days May Provide Heart Attack Protection, Science Daily news release <http://www.sciencedaily.com/releases/1998/12/981208133715.htm> retrieved Dec. 11, 1998

Forensic Science International (79,1:1)

Healthy Heart Handbook: Control Your Cholesterol, Lower Your Blood Pressure, and Clean Your Arteries — Naturally, FC&A Publishing, Peachtree City, Ga., 1999

International Journal of Epidemiology (15,3:326)

Journal of the American College of Cardiology (31,6:1226)

Medical Journal of Australia (155,11:757)

Psychology Today (31,6:20)

Psychosomatic Medicine (60,6:697)

Science News (155:70)

The Journal of the American Medical Association (277,20:1521 and 280,23:2001)

The New England Journal of Medicine (329,23:1677; 336,21:1473; 336,23:1678; and 339,19:1394)

This Week's Forecast May Be a Heart Attack, American Heart Association press release, Nov. 9, 1998

Heartburn

Archives of Family Medicine (4,8:718)

Medical Tribune for the Internist and Cardiologist (36,21:6 and 39,9:13)

Pharmacy Times (62,5:106)

Hemorrhoids

Diseases of the Colon and Rectum (38,5:453)

Drug Newsletter, Facts and Comparisons, St. Louis, Mo.

Emergency Medicine (25,8:19)

Environmental Nutrition (18,2:1)

Medical Update (18,2:3)

Modern Medicine (58,7:56)

Nature's Prescriptions: Foods, Vitamins, and Supplements That Prevent Disease, FC&A Publishing, Peachtree City, Ga., 1998

Postgraduate Medicine (92,2:141)

The Health Answer Book: The Complete Guide to Symptoms, Causes, and Natural Cures for Hundreds of Health Problems, FC&A Publishing, Peachtree City, Ga., 1997

Hiccups

Complete Guide to Symptoms, Illness & Surgery, The Body Press/Perigree Books, New York, 1989

Emergency Medicine (28,3:94)

Hiccups, Healthline Magazine <www.health-line.com> retrieved March, 26, 1999

The Lancet (338,8765:520)

The Physician and Sportsmedicine (23,5:18)

Your Good Health, Harvard University Press, Cambridge, Mass., 1987

High Blood Pressure

AMBI Nutrition Products: Cardia® Salt <http://www.ambiinc.com/nutrition/salt/cardia.html> retrieved Feb. 19, 1999

AMBI Nutrition Products: Clinical and Scientific Information About Cardia® Salt <http://www.ambiinc.com/nutrition/salt/cardia2.html> retrieved Feb. 19, 1999

American Journal of Hypertension (8,12:1184)

British Medical Journal (309,6952:436)

Caffeine <http://www.halifax.cbc.ca/streetcents/habits/caffeine.html> retrieved June 24, 1997

Geriatrics (51,6:19)

How to Prevent High Blood Pressure, National Heart, Lung, and Blood Institute <http://www.nhlbi.nih.gov> retrieved June 18, 1999

Hypertension (30,2:150; 31,1:131; and 32,2:260)

Journal of Applied Physiology (85,1:154)

Paul K. Whelton, M.D., Dean of the School of Public Health, Tulane University, New Orleans

Postgraduate Medicine (100,4:75)

Potassium, Healthlink Online Resources <http://www.healthlink.com/au> retrieved June 22, 1999

The chemistry of caffeine and related products <http://www.seas.upenn.edu/~cpage/caffeine/FAQ1.html> retrieved March 20, 1998

The Doctor's Complete Guide to Vitamins and Minerals, Dell Publishing, New York, 1994

The Journal of the American Medical Association (277,20:1624)

The Lancet (352,9129:709)

UVB Phototherapy, Department of Dermatology, Waikato Hospital, Hamilton, New Zealand <http://www.dermnet.org.nz/dna.uvb/uvb.html> retrieved Feb. 26, 1999

Impotence

Archives of Sexual Behavior (25,4:341)

British Journal of Clinical Practice (48,3:133)

Informed Decisions: The Complete Book of Cancer Diagnosis, Treatment, and Recovery, American Cancer Society

International Journal of Impotence Research (9,3:155)

The Prostate Answer Book, FC&A Publishing, Peachtree City, Ga., 1998

Insomnia

American Nephrology Nurses Association (24,6:672)

Annals of Pharmacotherapy (32,6:680)

Journal of the American Geriatric Society (46,6:700)

Pharmacology, Biochemistry, and Behavior (32,4:1065)

Postgraduate Medicine (79,2:265)

Sleep and the Traveler, National Sleep Foundation, <www.sleepfoundation.org> retrieved April 21, 1999

Super LifeSpan, Super Health, FC&A Publishing, Peachtree City, Ga., 1997

The Enchanted World of Sleep, Yale University Press, New Haven, Conn., 1996

The Journal of the American Medical Association (281,11:991)

Irritable Bowel Syndrome

Journal of Gastroenterology (32,6:765)

Mayo Clinic Health Letter (17,2:4)

Nature's Prescriptions: Foods, Vitamins and Supplements that Prevent Disease, FC&A Publishing, Peachtree City, Ga., 1998

The Complete German Commission E Monographs, Therapeutic Guide to Herbal Medicines, American Botanical Council, Austin, Texas, 1998

The Lancet (352,9135:1187)

Leg Pain

FDA Orders Stop to Marketing of Quinine for Night Leg Cramps, Food and Drug Administration Updates <www.verity.fda.gov> retrieved June 24, 1999

Natural Medicines and Cures Your Doctor Never Tells You About, FC&A Publishing, Peachtree City, Ga., 1996

The Health Answer Book, FC&A Publishing, Peachtree City, Ga., 1997

Tyler's Herbs of Choice: The Therapeutic Use of Phytomedicinals, The Haworth Herbal Press, Binghamton, N.Y., 1999

Lung Cancer

American Journal of Epidemiology (148,10:975)

Food, Nutraceuticals and Nutrition (22,11:2)

International Journal of Cancer (78,4:430)

Medical Tribune (39,9:13)

Mutation Research (402,1-2:307)

Natural Medicines and Cures Your Doctor Never Tells You About, FC&A Publishing, Peachtree City, Ga., 1995

Researchers discover how green tea may prevent cancer, Purdue University Health News (January 1999)

Super LifeSpan Super Health, FC&A Publishing, Peachtree City, Ga., 1997

Tufts University Health & Nutrition Letter (15,6:2)

Macular Degeneration

Eggs, American Heart Association, 7272 Greenville Ave., Dallas, TX 75231-4596

The British Journal of Ophthalmology (82,8:907)

Menopause

American Journal of Obstetrics and Gynecology (167,2:436)

Dr. Robert R. Freedman, Department of Obstetrics and Gynecology, Wayne State University, Detroit, Mich.

Constance Grauds, R.Ph., President of the Association of Natural Medicine Pharmacists, San Rafael, Calif.

Journal of Women's Health (7,9:1149)

Menopause: natural process or curable ailment?, Constance E. Grauds, R.Ph. <www.naturalland.com> retrieved April 26, 1999

Dr. Alice S. Rossi, Sociology Professor, University of Massachusetts, based on survey by the Research Network on Successful Midlife Development, sponsored by The John D. and Catherine T. MacArthur Foundation, conducted in 1995

Mitral Valve Prolapse Syndrome

American Heart Journal (129,1:83)

American Journal of Cardiology (79,6:768)

Journal of the American Dental Association (128,8:1142)

Mitral Valve Prolapse Treatment, Mitral Valve Prolapse Center, Birmingham, Ala. <http://www.mvprolapse.com/treat.htm> retrieved Jan. 6, 1999

Pacing and Clinical Electrophysiology (19,11[2]:1872)

Postgraduate Medicine (100,1:284)

Taking Control: Living With the Mitral Valve Prolapse Syndrome, Kardinal Publishing, Loveland, Ohio, 1996

The American Medical Association Encyclopedia of Medicine, Random House, Inc., New York, 1989

What is Dysautonomia? National Dysautonomia Research Foundation, P.O. Box 21153, Eagan, MN 55121-2553

Night Blindness

Fitoterapia (67,1:3)

New contacts looking up for over-50 set <www.thirdage.com/cgi-bin/NewsPrint.cg> retrieved Dec. 10, 1998

Over 60 Studies Link the Blue in Wild Blueberries to Health <www.wildblueberries.com> retrieved March 1, 1999

Wild Blueberry Association of North America, 59 Cottage St., P.O. Box 180, Bar Harbor, ME 04609

Wilhelmina Kalt, Ph.D., Food Chemist, Atlantic Food and Horticulture Research Center, Kentville, Nova Scotia, Canada

Osteoporosis

Alternative Medicine Digest (18:14)

Alternative Medicine Review (4,1:10)

Ann H. Hunt, Ph.D, Associate Professor of Nursing, Purdue University, West Lafayette, Ind.

Calcium: Important at Every Age, Texas Department of Health <www.tdh.state.tx.us> retrieved March 31, 1999

Canadian Space Agency news release (Oct. 29, 1998)

Exercise for Your Bone Health, Texas Department of Health <www.tdh.state.tx.us> retrieved March 31, 1999

Healthy Heart Handbook: Control Your Cholesterol, Lower Your Blood Pressure, and Clean Your Arteries — Naturally, FC&A Publishing, Peachtree City, Ga., 1999

Ipriflavone: The New Bone Builder, Nutrition Science News <www.nutritionsciencenews.com> retrieved April 6, 1999

Journal of the American College of Nutrition (15,6:553)

Nature's Prescriptions: Foods, Vitamins, and Supplements That Prevent Disease, FC&A Publishing, Peachtree City, Ga., 1998

Osteoporosis, American Academy of Orthopaedic Surgeons <www.aaos.org> retrieved March 31, 1999

Super LifeSpan, Super Health, FC&A Publishing, Peachtree City, Ga., 1997

The American Journal of Clinical Nutrition (68,6S:1364S and 69,1:74)

The Journal of the American Medical Association (272,24:1909)

The New England Journal of Medicine (335,16:1176)

Viactiv <http://www.viactic.com/produces/viactiv/productinfo.html> retrieved Feb. 24, 1999

Ovarian Cancer

American Journal of Epidemiology (130,3:497)

Cancer Epidemiology, Biomarkers and Prevention (5,9:733)

Journal of the National Cancer Institute (88,1:32)

Nutrition and Cancer (15,3-4:239)

What Every Woman Should Know About Ovarian Cancer, National Ovarian Cancer Coalition Ovarian Cancer Fact Sheet <http://www.ovarian.org> retrieved March 31, 1999

Ovarian Cancer Controversy: When and How To Use Available Screening Methods, Medscape Women's Health <http://www.medscape.com> retrieved March 31, 1999

Ovarian Cancer: Screening, Treatment, and Followup, National Institutes of Health Consensus Development Conference Statement <http://text.nlm.nih.gov> retrieved March 31, 1999

Study Shows Increased Risks of Ovarian Cancer, University of California, Irvine <http://www.newswise.com> retrieved March 25, 1999

Prostate Cancer

Cancer Causes and Controls (9,6:553)

Doctor Shopping: How to Choose the Right Doctor for You and Your Family, Health Information Press, Los Angeles, 1996

Hal Alpiar, President and CEO, Businessworks, Point Pleasant, N.J.

Journal of the National Cancer Institute (90,6:440; 90,16:1219; and 90,21:1637)

Proceedings of the National Academy of Sciences (95,8:4589)

Who's Who in Health Care, National Institute on Aging Information Center, P.O. Box 8057, Gaithersburg, MD 20898-8057

Raynaud's Phenomenon

Angiology (46,1:1 and 46,7:603)

Annals of Internal Medicine (129,3:208)

Archives of Dermatology (119,5:396)

Arthritis Today (11,6:8)

British Medical Journal (314,7081:644)

Cayenne, David L. Hoffman, M.N.I.M.H.
<http://www.healthy.net/library/books/hoffman/materiamedica/cayenne.h
tm> retrieved Jan. 26, 1999

Digestive Diseases and Sciences (43,8:1641)

Journal of Rheumatology (12,5:953)

Journal of the Southern Orthopaedic Association (5,1:37)

*Nipple vasospasm — a manifestation of Raynaud's phenomenon and a pre-
ventable cause of breastfeeding failure*
<http://www.gp.org.au/cls/raynaud.html> retrieved Jan. 6, 1999

Scandinavian Journal of Rheumatology (25,3:143)

Super LifeSpan, Super Health, FC&A Publishing, Peachtree City, Ga.,
1997

The American Medical Association Encyclopedia of Medicine, Random
House, Inc., New York, 1989

Vascular Medicine (2,4:296)

Sinusitis

American Family Physician (53,3:877)

American Journal of Rhinology (11,5:399)

Emergency Medicine (28,5:118)

European Journal of Medical Research (3,8:367)

FDA Consumer (26,8:20)

Mother Earth News (160:38)

Otolaryngology: Head & Neck Surgery (113,1:104)

Salt water rinse may prevent colds <www.dailynews.yahoo.com> retrieved
Sept. 22, 1998

*Sinus Survival: A Self-Help Guide for Allergies, Bronchitis, Colds, and
Sinusitis*, Jeremy P. Tarcher, Inc., Los Angeles, Calif., 1988

The Big Book of Health Tips, FC&A Publishing, Peachtree City, Ga., 1996

Skin Cancer

American Family Physician (49,1:91)

British Medical Journal (310,6984:912 and 312,7047:1621)

Cancer Causes and Controls (7,4:458)

Cancer Facts & Figures — 1995, American Cancer Society, 1599 Clifton Road N.E., Atlanta, Ga. 30329–4251

Cutis (56,6:313)

FDA Consumer (29,6:10)

Medical Tribune for the Internist and Cardiologist (35,1:2; 36,5:19; and 37,2:11)

Medical Update (14,10:1)

Natural Medicine (4,3:321)

Natural Medicines and Cures Your Doctor Never Tells You About, FC&A Publishing, Peachtree City, Ga., 1995

Nature Medicine (3,5:510)

Public Health Reports (108,2:176)

Reducing Your Risk of Skin Cancer, American Institute for Cancer Research, 1759 R Street, N.W., Washington, D.C. 20069

Skin Care and Aging, National Institute on Aging Age Page <www.nih.gov/nia/health/pubpub/skin> retrieved July 7, 1998

Sunscreen Drug Products for Over-the-Counter Human Use, Monograph, Part III, Federal Register, Department of Health and Human Services, Food and Drug Administration (58,90:28242)

Sunscreen Ingredient Causes DNA Damage in Light, American Chemical Society news release, Dec. 12, 1998

Sunscreens Miss Many Harmful Rays <www.msnbc.com/news> retrieved Sept. 1, 1998

The Health Answer Book: The Complete Guide to Symptoms, Causes, and Natural Cures for Hundreds of Health Problems, FC&A Publishing, Peachtree City, Ga., 1997

The Atlanta Journal/Constitution (Dec. 16, 1998, F3)

Stress

American Journal of Public Health (87,6:957 and 88,10:1469)

Breathing FAQ — Frequently Asked Questions
<www.breathing.com/faq.htm> retrieved Feb. 3, 1999

Conscious Breathing: Breathwork for Health, Stress Release, and Personal Mastery, Bantam Books, New York, 1995

European Heart Journal (19,11:1648)

Gay Hendricks, Ph.D., The Hendricks Institute, Santa Barbara, Calif.

Journal of Family Practice (39,4:349)

Medical schools to examine role of religion, Maranatha Christian Journal
<http://www.pe.net/mcj/news/news2268.htm> retrieved Jan. 11, 1999

Preventive Medicine (27,4:545)

Psychosomatic Medicine (57,1:5)

Social Science and Medicine (29,1:69)

Super LifeSpan, Super Health, FC&A Publishing, Peachtree City, Ga., 1997

The Big Book of Health Tips, FC&A Publishing, Peachtree City, Ga., 1996

Stroke

Brain Basics: Preventing Stroke, National Institute of Neurological Disorders and Stroke, National Institutes of Health, Bethesda, MD 20892

Circulation (98,12:1198)

Emergency Medicine (28,11:78)

Journal of Oral and Maxillofacial Surgery (56,8:950)

National Stroke Association <www.stroke.org/Press_Releases/980811-self-screen.html> retrieved March 18, 1999

Stroke (29,5:900; 29,9:1806; 29,10:2049; 29,12:2467; and 30,1:1)

The Journal of the American Medical Association (280,22:1930)

The Lancet (349,9059:1150)

TMJ

American Family Physician (49,7:1617)

Bruxism: A Fact Sheet for Patients, Academy of General Dentistry <http://www.nysagd.org/bruxism/htm> retrieved April 29, 1999

Tooth and Gum Disease

Adult Oral Health, Oral Health Information, ADHA Online <www.adha.org> retrieved March 23, 1999

Cosmetic Techniques, American Dental Association <www.ada.org> retrieved March 23, 1999

Current News Relevant to Dentistry, Joel B. Schilling, D.D.S. <http://idt.net/~jjjss/itn.html> retrieved March 23, 1999

Journal of Behavioral Medicine (3,3:233)

Journal of Clinical Dentistry (8,6:159)

Journal of Clinical Periodontology (23,9:873; 24,2:115; and 24,4:260)

Journal of the California Dental Association (26,3:186)

Journal of the Canadian Dental Association (64,5:357)

Keeping a Healthy Mouth: Tips for Older Adults, American Dental Association <www.ada.org> retrieved March 23, 1999

Natural Medicines and Cures Your Doctor Never Tells You About, FC&A Publishing, Peachtree City, Ga., 1995

Newsday (12:224 and PSA-2277)

Senior Oral Health, ADHA Online <www.adha.org> retrieved March 23, 1999

Taking Care of Your Teeth and Mouth, National Institute on Aging Age Page <www.aoa.dhhs.gov> retrieved March 23, 1999

The Truth About Tooth Whitening/Tooth Bleaching Systems, The Dental Zone <www.saveyoursmile.com> retrieved March 23, 1999

Tommy Turkiewicz, D.M.D., Peachtree City, Ga.

What To Do About Sensitive Teeth, The Dental Zone <www.saveyoursmile.com> retrieved March 23, 1999

Your Diet and Dental Health, American Dental Association <www.ada.org> retrieved March 23, 1999

Ulcers

Journal of Applied Bacteriology (73,5:388)

Journal of Pharmacy and Pharmacology (43,12:817)

Nature's Prescriptions: Foods, Vitamins, and Supplements That Prevent Disease, FC&A Publishing, Peachtree City, Ga., 1998

Warts

Miracle Healing Foods, Prentice Hall, Paramus, N.J., 1999

Plastic and Reconstructive Surgery (68,6:975)

The Medical Advisor: the Complete Guide to Alternative and Conventional Treatments, Time-Life Books, Alexandria, Va., 1996

Warts, American Academy of Dermatology, 930 N. Meachum Road, P.O. Box 4014, Schaumburg, IL 60168-4014

Weight Control

American Journal of Public Health (87,5:747)

Annals of Internal Medicine (130,6:471)

Clinical Cardiology (11,9:597)

Dieting and Gallstones, NIH Publication No. 94-3677, National Institute of Diabetes and Digestive and Kidney Diseases, 9000 Rockville Pike, Bethesda, MD 20892

Dr. Richard Mattes, Professor of Foods and Nutrition, Purdue University

Hamilton and Whitney's Nutrition Concepts and Controversies, West Publishing, St. Paul, Minn., 1994

Human Nutrition, Mosby, St. Louis, 1995

International Journal of Obesity and Related Metabolic Disorders (19,S7:S8)

International Journal of Sports Medicine (6,1:41)

Jerusalem artichoke may help ward off cancer, Minneapolis/St. Paul CityBusiness <http://www.amcity.com:80/twincities/stories/092898/story8.html> retrieved Sept. 28, 1998

Journal of Applied Psychology (83,6:944)

Journal of Gerontology (47,4:M99)

Journal of the American College of Nutrition (16,5:423)

Lenore S. Greenstein, Registered Dietitian, Naples, Florida

Medicine and Science in Sports and Exercise (17,4:456)

Metabolism (43,5:621)

New Tomato Breeding Lines Pack in Beta Carotene, U.S. and World News <www.sddt.com/files/librarywire/98/11/03/ch.html> retrieved March 11, 1999

Physiological Behavior (59,1:179)

Proceedings of the Society for Experimental Biology and Medicine (180,3:422)

Science (282,5396:2098 and 283,5399:212)

Strong Women Stay Young, Bantam Books, New York, 1998

The American Journal of Clinical Nutrition (51,3:428; 66,4:860 and 66,5:1110)

The Health Answer Book: A Complete Guide to Symptoms, Causes, and Natural Cures for Hundreds of Health Problems, FC&A Publishing, Peachtree City, Ga., 1997

The Journal of the American Medical Association (273,6:503)

The New Mighty Maroon Carrot, Texas Neighbors <http://165.91.48.7/vic/Press%20Release/new_mighty_maroon_carrot_.htm> retrieved March 11, 1999

The Obesity Factor, American Institute for Cancer Research Newsletter <www.aicr.org> retrieved Feb. 25, 1999

Index

Wine, for arthritis 26-27
Witch hazel 150, 214

Y

Yoga 70-75, 164
Yohimbine 226

Z

Zinc
  Alzheimer's disease and 15
  for BPH 154
  for colds 97
  for diabetes 119
  for impotence 224